THE COMPLETE DIABETES FOOD ENCYCLOPEDIA

OVER 4000+ FOODS RANKED BY GI, GL, NET CARBS & MEDITERRANEAN DIET COMPATIBILITY

DR. H. MAHER

❀ Created with Vellum

CONTENTS

INTRODUCTION

Living with Type 1 or Type 2 Diabetes can be daunting. It presents questions like, "What can I eat?" and "How can I prevent devastating complications such as Chronic Kidney Disease (CKD)?" But imagine having a powerful tool, a single, comprehensive resource that eases this journey by providing robust, reliable information rooted in the latest scientific research - a tool that not only aids in managing diabetes but also aids in preventing or slowing the progression of related complications. Welcome to "The Complete Diabetes Food Encyclopedia."

What sets this encyclopedia apart is its all-in-one, comprehensive approach to diabetes management. With an expansive food list that includes both diabetes-friendly options and those that should be avoided, it guides you in making informed dietary decisions. In-depth analysis and ratings for each food item are provided, covering aspects like Glycemic Load (GL), net carbohydrates, fats, and sodium content.

In addition to the detailed food analysis, this guide also incorporates meal planning strategies and practical application tips. You are not simply given data but taught how to use it to enhance your daily dietary decisions. These features are coupled with the principles of the trusted Mediterranean diet, aligning with the latest 2020-2025 Dietary Guidelines for Americans and the latest health and nutrition research findings.

This is not merely an informational book; it's an empowering tool that brings hope to those living with diabetes. The information is designed to be accessible and practical, facilitating your journey towards improved health. As you flip through the pages, you'll realize that better blood glucose control and a greater degree of freedom from the constraints of diabetes is within your reach. It's not about strict rules and limitations, but about understanding your choices and feeling empowered to make the best decisions for your health.

No doubt, diabetes presents challenges. But with "The Complete Diabetes Food Encyclopedia," you're not navigating the journey alone. This resource is a beacon of guidance, enlightening your path to a healthier life. Your transformation begins here. Are you ready to embrace it? Welcome to a new chapter of your life with diabetes. Welcome to a life of balance, wellness, and vitality.

A DEEPER DIVE INTO "THE COMPLETE DIABETES FOOD ENCYCLOPEDIA"

The real value of "The Complete Diabetes Food Encyclopedia" is in its comprehensive and detailed approach to diabetes management. This guide doesn't merely list food items—it distills complex dietary concepts into an easily navigable format, offering both broad and in-depth perspectives. Its unique features place it at the forefront of diabetes management resources:

Practical Organization and Accessibility: The encyclopedia is meticulously structured with an A-Z food list, allowing easy access to comprehensive information. This ensures that whether you're a healthcare provider, newly diagnosed with diabetes, or someone aiming to improve your dietary habits, you'll have a seamless navigation experience.

Comprehensive Food Analysis: Each food item listed is thoroughly analyzed, with crucial nutritional aspects such as Glycemic Index (GI), Glycemic Load (GL), net carbohydrates, fats, and sodium content detailed. This allows you to better understand the impact of your food choices on blood glucose levels and overall health, fostering informed decision-making.

Compliance Analysis with DiabeteBalance Diet Principles: The DiabeteBalance Diet, a critical component of this Encyclopedia, is a uniquely designed eating approach, fundamentally grounded in the best aspects of the Mediterranean Diet, Glycemic Load principles, and up-to-date nutritional science. It combines the heart-healthy, varied, and balanced nature of the Mediterranean Diet with the blood sugar control strategies of the Glycemic Load, providing a comprehensive and effective dietary strategy for managing diabetes.

Beyond simply listing nutritional facts, the Food List in this Encyclopedia also includes a robust compliance analysis with the principles of the DiabeteBalance Diet. This feature provides readers with a clear understanding of why specific foods are categorized as compliant or non-compliant. It bolsters the readers' ability to make educated dietary choices tailored to their individual health goals, thereby demystifying the often confusing world of diabetes-friendly foods.

This approach ensures the reader fully understands the diet before exploring how the principles are applied in practice. The food items, their analysis, and their compliance with the DiabeteBalance Diet are all interconnected aspects that provide a complete picture of managing diabetes through diet.

Connection with Real-life Scenarios: Bridging the gap between theory and practice, the encyclopedia offers practical guidance on incorporating these foods into daily meals. It provides detailed meal planning, portion size recommendations for each food, and explores the underlying principles of the DiabeteBalance Diet, turning nutritional insights into actionable steps.

Emphasis on Overall Health and Well-being: Beyond diabetes management, the guide promotes a holistic approach to health. By aligning with the principles of the Mediterranean Diet and the latest Dietary Guidelines, it encourages a balanced and nutritious eating pattern beneficial to everyone, not just those with diabetes.

This holistic approach is why "The Complete Diabetes Food Encyclopedia" stands apart—it doesn't merely present information, it provides context, promotes understanding, and guides practical application. Its evidence-based, approachable content empowers you to take control of your health, making diabetes management less daunting and more achievable.

PART I
UNDERSTANDING DIABETES:
A COMPREHENSIVE GUIDE

INSULIN: THE HORMONE'S ROLE

When being diagnosed with diabetes, or managing the condition, one term that frequently comes up is "insulin." Is it a drug, therapy, or hormone? How does it relate to diabetes, and why are terms like "insulin resistance" and "insulin sensitivity" important to understand, even when following therapy or a diet? This simplified overview will shed light on these questions and more.

What Is Insulin?

Insulin is a vital hormone produced and secreted by beta cells in the pancreas. It plays a critical role in stabilizing blood glucose levels in the body. Without it, our cells would be unable to effectively use glucose, a form of sugar that serves as the primary energy source. Insulin is neither a drug nor a therapy, but it is often used as a medication in insulin therapy for those with diabetes.

Insulin and Diabetes

Diabetes is a chronic illness where blood glucose levels become abnormally elevated. There are two main types:

- Type 1 Diabetes (T1D): The body's immune system attacks the beta cells that produce insulin, leading to little or no insulin production.

- Type 2 Diabetes (T2D): The body does become resistant to insulin, which means the cells do not respond effectively to insulin's actions. As a result, glucose from the bloodstream has difficulty entering the cells, leading to high blood glucose levels.

For individuals with T1D, insulin therapy becomes necessary to replace the hormone that the body no longer produces. In T2D, insulin therapy may be prescribed when other methods of controlling blood glucose are unsuccessful.

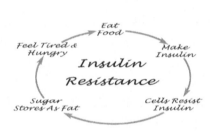

INSULIN RESISTANCE AND WHY YOU SHOULD CARE

Insulin resistance is a metabolic condition where the cells in the body become less responsive to the effects of insulin, the hormone responsible for regulating blood glucose levels. As a result, glucose has difficulty entering the cells, leading to higher blood glucose levels.

This impaired insulin response is a key factor in the development of T2D. Even if you diligently follow a specific diet or therapy, understanding and effectively managing insulin resistance are crucial to avoid potential complications.

Understanding and Managing Insulin Resistance

Insulin resistance is vital to recognize for effective diabetes control. It leads to reduced cellular response to insulin, requiring the pancreas to produce more insulin, resulting in various metabolic issues. This condition increases the risk of T2D, cardiovascular diseases, and other complications.

Epidemiology of Insulin Resistance

Insulin resistance is a rapidly growing global issue that impacts millions of people and is strongly linked to obesity and type 2 diabetes. Vulnerable populations include certain ethnic groups, older adults, and individuals with low socioeconomic status. Early intervention, focusing on adopting a healthy lifestyle, can effectively prevent or delay complications associated with insulin resistance.

Symptoms of Insulin Resistance

Insulin resistance, in its early stages, may often be asymptomatic. However, it can be indicated by skin disorders, weight gain, fatigue, polycystic ovary syndrome (PCOS), and hyperglycemia. If left untreated, it can progress and increase the risk of developing T2D, cardiovascular diseases, non-alcoholic fatty liver disease (NAFLD), PCOS, metabolic syndrome, sleep apnea, and neuropathy.

Complications of Insulin Resistance

Chronic insulin resistance can indeed lead to severe health issues, such as T2D, cardiovascular diseases, liver disorders, hormonal imbalances, metabolic syndrome, sleep disturbances, and nerve damage. However, adopting a healthy lifestyle and seeking appropriate medical interventions can effectively prevent or mitigate these complications.

Diagnosing Insulin Resistance

The diagnostic process involves conducting fasting blood glucose tests, OGTT, HbA1c test, HOMA-IR, and insulin sensitivity tests. Timely identification, along with lifestyle adjustments and, if needed, prescribed medication, are crucial for effective management.

INSULIN RESISTANCE IN PEOPLE WITH T2: IMPLICATIONS

Insulin resistance is a defining characteristic of T2D, and it's a condition that affects several crucial aspects of an individual's health. It's more than just an obstacle to blood glucose regulation; it also has significant implications for cardiovascular health, renal and nervous system functions, vision, and more. Further, it may exacerbate or contribute to other complications. It's therefore critical for those with type 2 diabetes to understand the broader impact of insulin resistance on their health, and how they can manage it effectively.

1. **Blood Glucose Management**: Insulin resistance is the main driver behind high blood sugar levels in type 2 diabetes. With insulin resistance, cells don't respond effectively to insulin's signals to take in glucose from the bloodstream. This leads to elevated blood sugar levels, or hyperglycemia, which can cause damage to various organs and tissues over time.

2. **Cardiovascular Health**: People with insulin resistance often have other comorbidities that raise the likelihood of heart disease and stroke, such as high blood pressure, abnormal cholesterol levels, and obesity. These factors collectively form a condition known as metabolic syndrome, which significantly increases cardiovascular risk.

3. **Kidney and Nerve Functions**: Chronic hyperglycemia caused by insulin resistance can damage the blood vessels in the kidneys, causing a condition known as diabetic nephropathy. It can also affect the nerves, leading to diabetic neuropathy, which can cause symptoms ranging from pain and numbness in the extremities to heart, blood vessels, digestive system, and urinary tract issues.

4. **Eye Health**: Elevated blood sugar levels can also harm the retina blood vessels leading to diabetic retinopathy. Poor

management diabetes can lead to vision loss, emphasizing the importance of early treatment.

To mitigate these risks and manage insulin resistance effectively, individuals with type 2 diabetes need to adopt a comprehensive approach that combines lifestyle modifications and, where necessary, medical treatment.

Medical Treatment: In some cases, lifestyle modifications may not be enough to manage insulin resistance. In these cases, your doctor may prescribe medication such as metformin, which can help improve insulin sensitivity. Working closely with your doctor to monitor blood sugar levels, adjust medications as necessary, and manage any side effects is important.

INSULIN SENSITIVITY: A POSSIBLE SOLUTION?

Enhanced insulin sensitivity enables the body's cells to efficiently utilize blood glucose, thereby reducing elevated blood sugar levels. On the other hand, low insulin sensitivity, commonly referred to as insulin resistance, can contribute to the development of type 2 diabetes and various health complications. Therefore, improving insulin sensitivity can be a critical step in managing diabetes and overall health.

Understanding Insulin Sensitivity:

Insulin is a hormone that acts like a key, allowing glucose (sugar) to enter cells from the bloodstream and be used for energy. Insulin sensitivity varies from person to person and is influenced by several factors, including diet, exercise, sleep, stress, and genetic factors. When your body is highly sensitive to insulin, less insulin is required to lower blood glucose levels. In contrast, insulin resistance is a state in which the body's cells do not respond adequately to insulin, inducing higher levels of insulin and glucose in the blood.

Role in Health and Disease:

High insulin sensitivity is generally associated with good health as it enables your body to regulate blood sugar levels efficiently. This not only helps to prevent high blood sugar and type 2 diabetes, but it also helps to maintain energy levels and prevent devastating diabetes complications. On the other hand, low insulin sensitivity (insulin resistance) increases the risk of chronic health problems and is associated with conditions like metabolic syndrome, obesity, heart and blood disease, and certain types of cancer.

Improving Insulin Sensitivity:

There are several strategies that can improve insulin sensitivity:

- **Diet**: Consuming a balanced diet that predominantly consists of whole, unprocessed foods can significantly enhance insulin sensitivity. Foods particularly high in fiber, such as whole grains, fruits, and vegetables, play a crucial role in regulating blood sugar levels effectively. Moreover, incorporating healthy fats, like those found in avocados, fatty fish, nuts, and seeds, along with lean proteins, can further contribute to maintaining insulin sensitivity at optimal levels.
- **Exercise**: Physical activity can increase insulin sensitivity because muscle contractions during exercise promote the cells' uptake of glucose, independently of insulin. Both aerobic exercise (like walking, running, and cycling) and resistance exercise (like weight lifting) have been shown to increase insulin sensitivity.
- **Weight Management**: Enhancing insulin sensitivity can be attained by maintaining a healthy weight or achieving weight loss if overweight. Even modest weight loss (5-10% of body weight) can have a consequent effect on insulin resistance.
- **Sleep and Stress Management**: Lack of sleep and chronic

8

stress can both worsen insulin sensitivity. Therefore, good sleep hygiene and stress management techniques, like meditation or yoga, can improve insulin sensitivity.

Insulin Sensitivity and Medical Treatment: Medications such as metformin can improve insulin sensitivity in people with type 2 diabetes or those at high risk of developing the disease. These drugs work by making the body's cells more responsive to insulin. However, they are typically used alongside lifestyle modifications, not as a substitute.

By understanding the concept of insulin sensitivity and implementing strategies to improve it, individuals can effectively manage their blood glucose levels, reduce their likelihood of developing T2D, and enhance their overall health.

UNDERSTANDING TYPE 2 DIABETES AND ITS MANAGEMENT

A COMPREHENSIVE HISTORY OF DIABETES

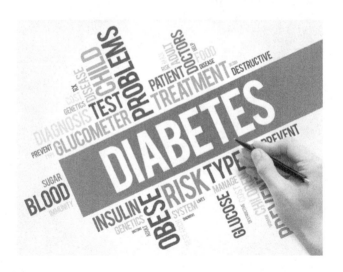

Diabetes, a chronic health condition characterized by the body's diffi-culty in regulating blood sugar levels, has a rich historical back-ground. Ancient civilizations such as the Egyptians, Indians, Chinese, and Greeks were among the first to recognize the signs of diabetes. They noticed that individuals with diabetes exhibited sweet-tasting urine, an observation that became a defining characteristic of the condition.

In the 1600s, an English physician named Thomas Willis officially coined the term "diabetes mellitus," which translates to "honey-sweet" in Latin, to describe this ailment.

The early 1900s marked a significant turning point in our understanding of diabetes when Canadian scientists Frederick Banting and Charles Best made a groundbreaking discovery. They identified insulin, a hormone secreted by the pancreas, responsible for facilitating the transport of sugar from the bloodstream into cells, where it is utilized for energy. This momentous breakthrough, which earned them the Nobel Prize in Physiology or Medicine in 1923, revolutionized the treatment of diabetes, particularly type 1 diabetes, where the body lacks sufficient insulin production.

Over time, researchers and medical experts delved deeper into the complexities of diabetes and identified various forms of the condition. Type 2 diabetes emerged as the most prevalent type, accounting for the majority of diabetes cases worldwide. It is characterized by the body's reduced sensitivity to insulin (insulin resistance) and inadequate insulin production. Another type is gestational diabetes, which affects some pregnant women and requires careful management to protect both the mother and the baby. Additionally, monogenic diabetes, caused by specific genetic mutations, represents a less common form.

In the realm of diabetes management, significant advancements have been made. Blood sugar level monitoring devices allow individuals to track their glucose levels regularly, aiding in better diabetes control. Insulin pumps offer a convenient and continuous way to deliver insulin, replacing the need for multiple injections. The development of improved forms of insulin with different action profiles has contributed to better glycemic control.

Lifestyle interventions have also been proven crucial in managing diabetes effectively. Healthy eating habits, physical activity, weight management, and blood pressure control are essential components of diabetes care. Moreover, patient education and support play a pivotal role in empowering individuals with T2D to take control of their health and make wise decisions about their diabetes management.

Despite these advancements, the prevalence of type 2 diabetes has been on the rise globally, largely driven by factors such as sedentary behavior, unhealthy dietary patterns, and increasing obesity rates. This alarming trend has prompted a greater emphasis on preventive efforts, early detection, and enhanced disease management.

HOW BLOOD SUGAR REGULATION WORKS IN HEALTHY INDIVIDUALS AND THOSE WITH TYPE 2 DIABETES

Blood sugar regulation in the human body is a meticulously orchestrated process to maintain glucose levels within a narrow range to ensure optimal cellular function. In healthy individuals, this process functions harmoniously, allowing the body to utilize glucose efficiently.

After consuming food, especially carbohydrates, the digestive system breaks down these complex molecules into glucose, which enters the bloodstream. When blood glucose levels increase, it prompts the pancreas beta cells to release insulin. Insulin acts as a key, unlocking the cell membranes to enable glucose entry into the cells, where it is utilized for energy production.

During periods between meals or fasting when blood glucose levels decrease, the pancreas releases the glucagon hormone. Glucagon signals the liver to convert its stored glycogen back into glucose, releasing it into the bloodstream to maintain stable blood sugar levels.

However, in type 2 diabetes, this intricate balance is disrupted. As cells become unsusceptible to the insulin effects, their ability to efficiently absorb glucose is impaired. Consequently, glucose accumulates in the bloodstream, resulting in hyperglycemia or high blood sugar levels. To compensate for the resistance, the pancreas produces and releases more insulin in an attempt to lower blood glucose levels. This prolonged hyperinsulinemia can further contribute to insulin resistance, creating a vicious cycle.

Furthermore, the liver's regulation of glucose production may be compromised, leading to increased glucose release into the bloodstream, exacerbating the hyperglycemic state.

Effective management of type 2 diabetes often involves addressing insulin resistance, restoring insulin sensitivity, and re-establishing normal blood sugar regulation.

INSULIN RESISTANCE AND THE ONSET OF T2D

Insulin resistance serves as a critical precursor to the development of type 2 diabetes. At this stage, cells, particularly those in the liver, muscles, and adipose tissue, become less responsive to the effects of insulin. As a result, glucose uptake into these cells is hindered, leading to elevated blood glucose levels.

In response to insulin resistance, the pancreas attempts to compensate by producing more insulin, leading to hyperinsulinemia. Initially, this compensatory mechanism helps maintain blood sugar levels within a relatively normal range. However, over time, the continuous demand for high insulin levels may overwhelm the beta cells of the pancreas, causing them to gradually lose their ability to produce sufficient insulin.

As the insulin-producing capacity of the pancreas declines, blood glucose levels start to rise, eventually reaching the range of prediabetes or overt type 2 diabetes. In prediabetes, blood glucose levels are above normal but not yet elevated enough to meet the criteria for a diabetes diagnosis. Without appropriate intervention, prediabetes can progress to full-fledged type 2 diabetes.

It is essential to emphasize that insulin resistance can be impacted by a variety of genetic predisposition and lifestyle factors. Being overweight or obese, sedentary habits, and unhealthy dietary patterns are significant contributors to insulin resistance and the development of type 2 diabetes.

DIAGNOSIS AND MANAGEMENT OF TYPE 2 DIABETES

The diagnosis of type 2 diabetes typically involves assessing blood sugar levels through various tests, enabling healthcare professionals to make an accurate assessment. Some of the commonly used tests for diagnosing and monitoring type 2 diabetes include:

- **Fasting Blood Sugar Test:** This test involves measuring blood glucose levels after an overnight fast (usually eight hours or more). A fasting blood sugar level higher or equal to 126 mg/dL (7.0 mmol/L) on two separate tests indicates diabetes.
- **HbA1c Test:** The HbA1c test provides an average blood sugar level over the past two to three months. An HbA1c level of 6.5% or higher is considered indicative of diabetes.
- **Oral Glucose Tolerance Test (OGTT):** During the OGTT, the individual consumes a sugary solution, and blood sugar levels are measured two hours later. A blood sugar level higher or equal to 200 mg/dL (11.1 mmol/L) indicates diabetes.
- **C-Peptide Test:** This test measures C-peptide, a byproduct of insulin production, to gauge insulin levels in the body. A C-peptide test helps distinguish between type 1 and type 2 diabetes. Low C-peptide levels may indicate reduced insulin production, suggesting type 1 diabetes. In contrast, elevated or normal C-peptide levels often suggest type 2 diabetes,

which is characterized by insulin resistance and relatively preserved insulin secretion.

Once diagnosed, the management of type 2 diabetes aims to achieve and maintain optimal blood sugar control, prevent complications, and enhance overall well-being. Diabetes management strategies encompass a multifaceted approach such as the DiabeteBalance Diet

RISK FACTORS

Type 2 Diabetes has various risk factors. Some, such as being overweight, obese, or vitamin D deficient, are controllable, while others like age and family history are not. Known risk factors include:

- **Overweight and obesity:** These are two main predictors of developing type 2 diabetes. However, they are reversible through an adequate diet, such as the glycemic load.
- **Type 2 diabetes family history:** The risk of developing T2DM increases if a parent or sibling has it.
- **Ethnicity:** T2DM is more prevalent in certain ethnic groups, including African American, Hispanic or Latino, American Indian, or Asian American.
- **Age 45 or older:** Although it generally occurs after the age of forty-five, it can develop earlier in life.
- **High blood pressure (hypertension):** High blood pressure can significantly raise the risk of developing T2DM and cardiovascular diseases.
- **Polycystic ovary syndrome (PCOS):** This condition has been identified as a risk factor due to its association with insulin resistance.
- **Vitamin D deficiency:** Poor vitamin D status is linked to increased risk for insulin resistance and/or metabolic

syndrome, though proper levels can improve insulin sensitivity and T2DM management.

SYMPTOMS OF TYPE 2 DIABETES

Type 2 diabetes may not cause noticeable symptoms in its early stages, allowing the condition to remain undiagnosed for an extended period. However, as blood sugar levels become persistently elevated, symptoms may gradually manifest. Common symptoms of type 2 diabetes include:

1. **Frequent Urination:** Increased thirst and frequent urination are common early signs of diabetes. Elevated blood sugar levels lead to the excretion of excess glucose through the urine.
2. **Unexplained Weight Loss:** Despite increased hunger and food intake, individuals with type 2 diabetes may experience unexplained weight loss due to the body's inability to properly utilize glucose for energy.
3. **Fatigue:** Persistently high blood sugar levels can lead to fatigue and a lack of energy.
4. **Blurred Vision:** Elevated blood sugar levels can result in temporary alterations in the shape of the eye lens, which may lead to vision blurriness.
5. **Slow-Healing Wounds:** Poorly controlled diabetes can impair wound healing and increase the risk of infections.
6. **Frequent Infections:** Diabetes can compromise the immune system, rendering individuals more vulnerable to infections, particularly urinary tract infections, skin infections, and yeast infections.
7. **Darkened Skin Patches:** Some individuals with diabetes may develop darkened, velvety patches of skin, a condition known

as acanthosis nigricans, usually in areas like the neck, armpits, or groin.

Identifying these symptoms and promptly seeking medical attention is vital for an accurate diagnosis and timely management.

TYPE 2 DIABETES COMPLICATIONS

Uncontrolled or poorly managed type 2 diabetes can lead to various complications affecting different organs and systems in the body:

- **Cardiovascular Complications:** High blood sugar levels can damage blood vessels, leading to atherosclerosis (narrowing and hardening of arteries) and an increased risk of heart disease, heart attacks, and strokes.
- **Neuropathy:** Persistently high blood sugar levels can lead to nerve damage, resulting in symptoms like numbness, tingling, pain, and weakness, often beginning in the feet and hands.
- **Nephropathy:** Diabetes can adversely affect the kidneys, leading to diabetic nephropathy. This condition may progress to chronic kidney disease, eventually requiring dialysis or kidney transplantation.
- **Immune Dysfunction:** Impaired immune function can make individuals with diabetes more susceptible to infections and slow down the healing process.
- **Ophthalmic Complications:** Damage to the small blood vessels in the eyes can lead to diabetic retinopathy, an illness that induce vision problems and even blindness if left untreated.
- **Peripheral Vascular Disease:** Inadequate blood flow to the extremities, particularly the feet, can result in peripheral vascular disease, elevating the risk of non-healing wounds, ulcers, and, in severe instances, the need for amputation.

- **Dental Problems:** Diabetes may contribute to dental problems like increased plaque formation, cavities, and gum disease.

Proper management of type 2 diabetes is essential to prevent, halt or delay these complications and maintain a good quality of life.

LIVING WITH TYPE 2 DIABETES: NAVIGATING THE PATH, UNDERSTANDING THE IMPACTS, AND SEEKING SOLUTIONS

Type 2 Diabetes (T2D) is a multifaceted condition that intertwines with various aspects of an individual's life. Living with T2D isn't just about grappling with high blood sugar levels. It's a broader narrative that spans understanding its genesis, making informed daily choices, and tapping into comprehensive solutions for a balanced life.

Challenges and Impacts:

Life with T2D presents its unique hurdles. Beyond the medical regimen, individuals grapple with lifestyle modifications, weight management issues, and potential societal misconceptions. The implications of these challenges can be profound.

Insulin Resistance: A primary hallmark of T2D, the body's decreased sensitivity to insulin, necessitates individuals to comprehend its dietary and lifestyle triggers and adjust accordingly.

Complications: Chronic and uncontrolled T2D has the potential to usher in a range of complications. These can encompass cardiovascular diseases, neuropathy, retinopathy, and renal issues, all bearing significant impacts on an individual's quality of life.

The DiabeteBalance Diet: A Beacon of Hope:

Within the tapestry of T2D management tools, the DiabeteBalance

Diet shines prominently. Crafted with precision, this dietary approach isn't merely a guideline for blood sugar control. It's a comprehensive blueprint for holistic health. It underscores the value of nutrient-dense foods, advocates for consistent glycemic control, and emphasizes the significance of individual dietary needs, fostering customization and adaptability.

In summation, living with T2D requires more than a reactive stance; it demands proactive engagement. With robust tools at their disposal, like the DiabeteBalance Diet, and a fortified support system, individuals with T2D can traverse their journey with confidence, leading lives marked by health, vitality, and empowerment.

UNDERSTANDING TYPE 1 DIABETES
AND ITS MANAGEMENT

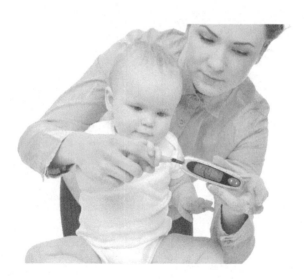

Type 1 diabetes (T1D) is a persistent autoimmune illness character-ized by the immune system's destruction of insulin-producing pancreatic *beta* cells. The body will no longer make insulin due to irreversible damage to the insulin-producing cells. Without insulin hormones, glucose can not get into the body's cells, and the blood glucose increases above normal. People with type 1 must inject daily insulin doses and follow a strict diet to stay alive and prevent severe adverse effects. Type 1 diabetes generally appears in children and young adults but may occur at any age.

In 2016, the FDA—Food and Drug Administration approved the artificial pancreas to replace manual blood glucose checking and the injection of insulin shots. These automated devices act like your real pancreas in controlling blood sugar and releasing insulin when the patient's blood sugar becomes too high. The artificial pancreas also releases a small flow of insulin continuously.

HOW BLOOD SUGAR REGULATION WORKS IN HEALTHY INDIVIDUALS AND THOSE WITH TYPE 2 DIABETES

Blood sugar regulation is vital for maintaining the body's overall health and energy balance. The process involves complex interactions between insulin, glucose, and other hormones. In people with Type 1 Diabetes (T1D), this regulation is profoundly affected. This chapter explores the intricacies of blood sugar regulation in healthy individuals and those with T1D.

Blood Sugar Regulation in Healthy Individuals

In an individual with good health, the pancreas secretes insulin, allowing cells to absorb glucose for energy. Glucagon, another hormone, helps to convert stored glycogen back to glucose to maintain stable blood sugar levels. Together, these processes ensure energy balance and proper bodily function.

Disruption of Blood Sugar Regulation in T1D

Unlike T2D, where cells become resistant to insulin, T1D is marked by the autoimmune destruction of insulin-producing cells in the pancreas. Without insulin, glucose cannot enter cells, leading to a rise in blood sugar levels.

THE ONSET OF TYPE 1 DIABETES

T1D often develops during childhood or adolescence. The destruction of insulin-producing cells may occur over weeks to years, resulting in a lack of insulin. Unlike T2D, lifestyle factors are not the main triggers for T1D. The onset can be influenced by a genetic predisposition and various environmental factors, such as viral infections.

Diagnosis and Management of Type 1 Diabetes

Diagnosing Type 1 Diabetes (T1D) is a comprehensive process that requires thorough testing to ensure accurate results. Differentiating between T1D and other forms of diabetes, particularly Type 2, is crucial for implementing the most appropriate management strategy. Utilizing a combination of diagnostic tests allows healthcare professionals to assess the exact nature of the diabetes present. These tests include:

- **Fasting Blood Sugar Test**: A blood sugar level equal to or exceeding 126 mg/dL is indicative of diabetes.
- **HbA1c Test**: A level of 6.5% or higher indicates the presence of diabetes.
- **C-Peptide Test**: This measures C-peptide, a byproduct of insulin production, to gauge insulin levels. A C-peptide test helps distinguish between type 1 and type 2 diabetes. Low C-peptide levels may indicate reduced insulin production, suggesting type 1 diabetes. In contrast, elevated or normal C-peptide levels often suggest type 2 diabetes, which is characterized by insulin resistance and relatively preserved insulin secretion.

STRATEGIES FOR MANAGING TYPE 1 DIABETES (T1D)

Type 1 Diabetes management is an intricate process that necessitates a multi-faceted approach. As the body ceases to produce insulin in T1D, individuals must incorporate a mix of treatments and lifestyle modifications to maintain their health. Here's a closer look at the core components of effective T1D management:

Insulin Therapy:

- **Rationale:** In T1D, the body's immune system destroys insulin-producing cells, leading to a lack of insulin. To compensate, exogenous insulin is required.
- **Methods:** Insulin can be administered through injections using syringes or insulin pens. Another approach is the use of insulin pumps that provide a continuous supply and allow for varied dosing.

Routine Monitoring:

- **Importance:** Regularly checking blood glucose levels is vital to verify they remain within the target range. It helps prevent complications, such as hypoglycemia (low blood sugar) or hyperglycemia (high blood sugar).
- **Methods:** Blood glucose meters provide immediate readings, while continuous glucose monitors (CGMs) offer real-time tracking of sugar levels throughout the day.

Balanced and Nutritious Diet:

- **Purpose:** Food intake directly impacts blood glucose levels. The DiabeteBalance diet ensures that the body receives necessary nutrients without causing extreme fluctuations in sugar levels.
- **Strategies:** Carbohydrate counting helps estimate the amount

of insulin required. Consuming low-glycemic index foods can lead to slower, more predictable changes in blood glucose. Regular consultation with your healthcare provider, coupled with the knowledge you'll gain from this book, will assist you in creating a personalized meal plan tailored to your specific needs and health goals.

Regular Exercise:

- **Benefits:** Physical activity helps improve insulin sensitivity, meaning the body can use insulin more efficiently. Additionally, exercise supports cardiovascular health, weight management, and overall well-being.
- **Considerations:** It's crucial to monitor blood sugar before, during, and after exercise. Some activities might require adjustments in insulin dosage or additional carbohydrate intake to prevent hypoglycemia.

While T1D poses challenges, with careful management and a holistic approach, you can lead healthy, fulfilling lives.

RISK FACTORS

Type 1 diabetes has diverse and complex risk factors. Some of these are still being explored, but key known risks include:

- **Family History**: Having a parent, brother, or sister diagnosed with T1D significantly raises the risk.
- **Ethnicity**: In the United States, white individuals are at higher risk compared to African American, Hispanic, or Latino people.
- **Age**: Although T1D typically occurs at an early age, it can

develop at any time. Its prevalence in teens and young adults is rising.

- **Viral Infections**: Viruses such as coxsackievirus B, mumps virus, and cytomegalovirus may trigger T1D by impacting the immune system.
- **Vitamin D Deficiency**: Inadequate vitamin D may increase T1D risk due to its essential role in immune system regulation.

SYMPTOMS OF TYPE 1 DIABETES

Symptoms of T1D can arise suddenly and may be severe. They include:

- Frequent thirst and urination
- Increased hunger
- Fruity-smelling breath, indicating diabetic ketoacidosis (DKA)
- Unexplained weight loss
- Blurred vision
- Stomach pains
- Nausea and vomiting
- Recurrent urinary infections
- Fatigue and tiredness

TYPE 1 DIABETES COMPLICATIONS

Poorly managed T1D can lead to serious complications, such as:

- **Blood Vessels and Heart**: Higher risk of heart diseases and stroke

- **Nerves**: Potential damage causing sensations like numbness and tingling
- **Kidneys**: Risk of damage leading to dialysis or transplant
- **Eyes**: Possibility of vision impairment or blindness
- **Feet**: Increased risk of injuries, ulcers, and even amputation
- **Immune System**: Elevated susceptibility to infections
- **Mental Health**: Greater likelihood of anxiety and depression

Proactive and ongoing blood sugar management, through insulin therapy and regular medical check-ups, is essential to prevent these complications.

LIVING WITH TYPE 1 DIABETES: CHALLENGES, STAKES, AND SOLUTIONS

Type 1 Diabetes is more than just a medical condition; it's a life journey riddled with challenges but also paved with opportunities for resilience, adaptation, and personal growth. Living with T1D goes beyond mere management of blood glucose levels. It's about understanding the complexities, embracing the lifestyle shifts, and seeking holistic approaches to health.

Challenges and Stakes: Daily life with T1D introduces its unique set of challenges. From navigating dietary choices, managing stress, and adjusting insulin dosages, to understanding the impact of physical activity, individuals with T1D must become proactive partners in their healthcare. The stakes are high. Inconsistent or imprecise management can lead to complications, both immediate and long-term.

Hypoglycemia: One of the more immediate concerns for T1D individuals is hypoglycemia, a condition where blood sugar drops to dangerously low levels, leading to symptoms like confusion, dizziness, and in severe cases, unconsciousness.

Complications: Long-term mismanagement or uncontrolled T1D can lead to a host of complications. This includes cardiovascular issues, nerve damage, kidney problems, and eye complications, to name a few.

The DiabeteBalance Diet: Part of the Solution:

Amid these challenges, solutions emerge. A cornerstone among them is the DiabeteBalance Diet. This tailored approach to nutrition is not just about maintaining optimal blood glucose levels but also about supporting overall well-being. It emphasizes nutrient-rich foods, promotes balanced glycemic responses, and recognizes the individuality of every T1D patient, allowing for personalization and adaptability.

In essence, living with T1D is a balancing act—one that requires awareness, education, and a proactive stance. With the right tools, support, and dietary approaches like the DiabeteBalance Diet, individuals with T1D can navigate the challenges and lead a life defined not by their condition but by their determination and zest for life.

GESTATIONAL DIABETES MELLITUS (GDM): A COMPREHENSIVE UNDERSTANDING

Gestational diabetes (GDM) is a unique form of diabetes that specifically occurs during pregnancy in women without a prior history of the condition. Typically manifesting in the second or third trimester, GDM can, however, arise at any point during pregnancy and generally resolves postpartum. Nevertheless, it does predispose women to an increased likelihhod of developing type 2 diabetes in the future, particularly if accompanied by other risk factors such as obesity, imbalanced diet, a sedentary lifestyle, and metabolic syndrome.

PREVALENCE, SEVERITY, AND PATHOGENESIS

GDM affects between 2% and 10% of pregnancies globally, a variation stemming from differences in populations and diagnostic criteria. The condition's severity varies widely among individuals, ranging from mild to severe, depending on the blood glucose levels and accompanying complications.

The pathogenesis of gestational diabetes remains partly unknown but is thought to be associated with hormonal shifts during pregnancy that impede insulin utilization. Contributing factors to GDM include insulin resistance caused by placental hormones and pancreatic beta-cell dysfunction, resulting in insufficient insulin production to overcome resistance. Additional risk factors encompass family history of diabetes, obesity, and previous gestational diabetes episodes.

SYMPTOMS AND DIAGNOSIS

Most cases of gestational diabetes are asymptomatic, often slipping under the radar. When symptoms do occur, they may be mistaken for typical pregnancy discomfort. These symptoms parallel those of type 2 diabetes and may include:

- Intense thirst
- Increased hunger
- Unusual fatigue
- Stomach pains
- Nausea and vomiting
- Frequent urination
- Urinary infections
- Headaches

Routine prenatal screening tests typically conducted between the 24th and 28th weeks of pregnancy often detect the condition.

TREATMENT AND MANAGEMENT

The primary therapeutic objective for GDM is to regulate blood glucose levels during pregnancy to safeguard the wellbeing of both mother and child. Management strategies encompass:

Dietary Modifications: Emphasizing whole grains, lean proteins, and abundant fruits and vegetables.

Physical Activity: To augment insulin sensitivity and diminish blood glucose levels.

Self-Monitoring: Regular monitoring of blood glucose levels to ensure adherence to target ranges.

Insulin Therapy: In some instances, insulin may be necessary to control blood glucose levels.

Complications and Future Risks

If mismanaged, GDM can amplify the risk of complications for both mother and child, including:

- **Macrosomia**: Excessive fetal growth leading to delivery complications.
- **Preeclampsia**: A grave condition marked by high blood pressure and organ damage.
- **Neonatal Hypoglycemia**: Which may necessitate intervention.
- **Future Type 2 Diabetes**: For the mother, the risk is heightened.

Most women with GDM experience a reversal of the condition after childbirth. However, ongoing blood sugar monitoring is crucial, given the substantial risk of subsequent type 2 diabetes development among this demographic. Collaborative care involving healthcare providers, dietitians, and diabetes educators can optimize outcomes and reduce risks associated with GDM.

Through comprehending the risk factors, recognizing the symptoms, exploring available treatment options, and being aware of potential complications linked with gestational diabetes, women can proactively manage their condition and diminish the likelihood of complications. This approach ensures the well-being of both the mother and the developing baby.

MANAGING LOW BLOOD SUGAR

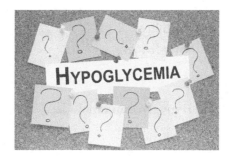

BLOOD GLUCOSE AND HYPOGLYCEMIA

Blood glucose levels fluctuate throughout the day. A level below 70 mg/dL is referred to as hypoglycemia or low blood sugar. This condition is common among those with both type 1 and type 2 diabetes, specifically those undergoing drug therapies such as insulin or other diabetes medications.

Hypoglycemia requires urgent action to restore blood sugar levels. Severe hypoglycemia can escalate into a diabetic emergency, making self-treatment impossible and necessitating assistance. Understanding its causes, signs, and symptoms is vital for prompt and effective treatment.

SYMPTOMS OF HYPOGLYCEMIA

Most individuals with diabetes exhibit symptoms when their blood sugar falls to 70 mg/dL or lower. Though unwelcome, these symptoms signal the body's need for carbohydrate intake to correct low blood sugar.

Mild-to-Moderate Symptoms include:

- Fast or irregular heartbeat
- Shaking
- Abnormal sweating
- Anxiety
- Nervousness or irritability
- Dizziness and lightheadedness
- Hunger

Symptoms of Severe Hypoglycemia include:

- Loss of consciousness
- Confusion and disorientation
- Difficulty concentrating
- Behavioral changes (e.g., nervousness, irritability, anxiety)
- Convulsions or seizures
- Coma

WHAT LEADS TO LOW BLOOD GLUCOSE IN INDIVIDUALS WITH DIABETES?

Various factors can lead to low blood sugar, including:

- **Over-medication:** Taking too much insulin or medicines that stimulate insulin release.
- **Dietary Mismanagement:** Insufficient carbohydrate consumption, meal delays, or skipping meals, especially when taking insulin or certain drugs.
- **Fasting:** Especially risky while on insulin or glucose-lowering drugs.
- **Excessive Exercise:** Strength training with low carbohydrate intake may cause sudden insulin drops.
- **Weather Conditions:** Hot and humid weather can enhance insulin absorption, raising hypoglycemia risk.
- **Alcohol Consumption:** Especially with heavy drinking and specific medications, the liver may not release enough glycogen to maintain blood sugar levels.

Hypoglycemia Unawareness

This condition occurs when a person does not notice hypoglycemia symptoms. Regular blood sugar checks or continuous glucose monitoring (CGM) devices may be necessary to detect and address low levels promptly.

PREVENTING HYPOGLYCEMIA

For those with diabetes, prevention is key:

- **Regular Monitoring:** Follow your healthcare provider's guidance on checking blood sugar levels.

- **Meal Planning:** Stick to a consistent schedule and balanced meal composition.
- **Medication Management:** Adhere to prescribed insulin or medication dosages.
- **Exercise Management:** Monitor and adjust carbohydrate intake and insulin around physical activities.

HOW TO TREAT LOW BLOOD SUGAR?

Immediate action is essential, as untreated hypoglycemia can be life-threatening.

The 15-15 Rule: For levels between 55-69 mg/dL, consume 15 to 20 grams of fast-acting carbohydrates and reverify your blood sugar after 15 minutes. Repeat if necessary, followed by a nourishing snack or meal.

Sources for 15 to 20 grams of carbohydrate include:

- 3 teaspoons of sugar, honey, or corn syrup
- 3 glucose tablets
- 1/2 cup (4 oz) of fruit juice or regular soda
- One slice of bread, small banana, medium apple, regular yogurt, 20 grapes
- 1/2 cup of cooked couscous or pasta
- 1 cup of milk (8 oz)

Treating Severe Hypoglycemia

This critical condition requires intervention by others, using glucagon—a prescribed hormone to raise blood sugar levels. There are nasal and injectable forms. Ensure those around you know how to recognize severe hypoglycemia, administer glucagon, and where to find it.

PART II
KNOWING WHAT'S IN THE
FOOD YOU EAT

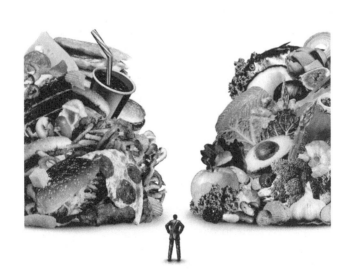

THE WESTERN DIET: A PATTERN OF CONCERN

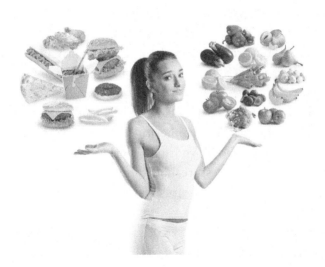

The Western diet, prevalent in many developed nations, has become a topic of significant concern among health professionals and researchers. This dietary pattern, characterized by high consumption of red and processed meats, sugary desserts, high-fat foods, refined grains, high-fat dairy products, sugary drinks, and excessive sodium, has contributed to an array of health complications. It's a diet that emphasizes processed and calorie-dense foods while often neglecting essential nutrients found in raw fruits, raw vegetables, whole grains, and lean proteins.

EFFECTS ON HEALTH

Over the years, the energy density of the Western diet has escalated, with alarming associations with various health issues:

- **Obesity:** The calorie-dense nature of this diet, coupled with low nutritional value, has been a leading factor in the global rise of obesity. Excessive calorie intake without adequate nutrient content leads to weight gain and obesity-related health problems.
- **Type 2 Diabetes:** This dietary pattern contributes to insulin resistance, a primary factor in the development and progression of T2D. Regular consumption of sugary and refined carbohydrate-rich foods can lead to chronic elevation of blood sugar levels, increasing the risk of developing diabetes.
- **Metabolic Disorders:** An imbalance in nutrients and excessive consumption of unhealthy fats and sugars can contribute to metabolic syndrome, a group of conditions that involve high blood pressure, high blood sugar, and abnormal cholesterol levels. These factors elevate the risk of heart disease, stroke, and diabetes.
- **Heart Disease:** High levels of saturated fats, trans fats, and sodium are linked to increased cholesterol levels and hypertension, leading to an increased risk of heart disease and cardiovascular events.
- **Cancers:** Diets high in processed meats and low in fiber have been associated with various cancers, including colon cancer. The chemicals and preservatives in processed meats, combined with the lack of protective nutrients from fruits and vegetables, contribute to this risk.

The Connection to Diabetes Management

The Western diet's impact on glucose metabolism and insulin sensitivity makes it a subject of concern in diabetes management. The high glycemic index of many foods within this diet leads to rapid spikes in blood sugar, complicating the control of diabetes. The excess of unhealthy fats may further deteriorate insulin sensitivity, making blood sugar management more challenging.

THE DIABETEBALANCE DIET: A COUNTERACTIVE APPROACH

Given the detrimental health effects of the Western diet, a substantial shift towards healthier, balanced eating is not merely advisable but essential. The DiabeteBalance Diet is proposed as a response to this challenge.

- **Nutrient Focus:** This diet emphasizes the consumption of nutrient-rich foods often lacking in the Western diet, such as raw vegetables, raw fruits, whole grains, and lean proteins. These foods provide essential vitamins, minerals, and dietary fiber, promoting better blood sugar control and overall health.
- **Portion Control:** Managing portion sizes helps in weight control, an essential aspect of diabetes management. By controlling portion sizes, individuals can better manage their calorie intake and prevent excessive blood sugar fluctuations.
- **Regular Physical Activity:** Exercise is encouraged to enhance insulin sensitivity and improve overall health. Regular physical exercise aids the body utilize glucose more effectively, reducing the need for higher insulin levels.
- **Consistent Meal Timing:** Regular and balanced meal times aid in maintaining stable blood sugar levels. Consistency in meal timing helps the body anticipate nutrient intake, allowing for better blood sugar regulation.
- **Gradual Transition:** Gradually shifting from the calorie-

dense Western diet to the nutrient-focused DiabeteBalance Diet can lead to effective management of diabetes. Slowly adopting healthier eating habits increases the likelihood of long-term success in managing diabetes.

- **Emphasizing Healthy Fats:** Reducing the intake of trans and saturated fats and incorporating healthy fats like omega-3 fatty acids support heart health, a vital consideration for people with diabetes. Healthy fats can help lower inflammation and improve cholesterol levels.

The Western diet's pattern presents genuine risks and challenges, particularly in diabetes management. By embracing principles such as those found in the DiabeteBalance Diet, individuals can undertake a transformative lifestyle change. This shift is not merely a temporary fix but a long-term solution aimed at enhancing overall well-being and combating chronic diseases, especially diabetes. Health professionals must engage in patient education and support to facilitate this essential dietary transition, promoting a comprehensive approach to wellness and disease prevention. Through collective efforts to promote healthier eating habits and regular physical activity, we can make significant strides in reducing the prevalence and impact of diabetes and related health conditions in society.

CARBOHYDRATES IN THE WESTERN DIET: A COMPLEX PICTURE

Carbohydrates play a significant role in the Western diet, encompassing both complex forms like starch and simple sugars such as sucrose, lactose, and fructose. Simple sugars have become a predominant part of the Western diet due to their inclusion in sugary drinks, highly processed foods, candies, and baked goods. The consumption of these sugars can cause rapid spikes in blood sugar levels, resulting in raised insulin production. Over time, this may contribute to insulin resistance, a precursor to T2D, and elevate cortisol levels, a stress hormone that can further imbalance blood sugar regulation.

In addition, this dietary pattern often lacks sufficient microbiota-accessible carbohydrates (MACs), which are essential for maintaining a healthy gut microbiota community. Inadequate MACs can result in reduced microbial diversity and a decline in the production of short-chain fatty acids (SCFAs), potentially impacting overall health. Specifically, the lack of MACs can impair insulin sensitivity, thereby complicating diabetes management and increasing the risk of other metabolic disorders.

Typically, the Western diet involves consuming 200-300 grams of carbohydrates per day. Hidden sugars are often overlooked; even salty preparations and beverages can contain surprising amounts of sugar, contributing to the overall carbohydrate load. While carbohydrates serve as a vital energy source for the body, this high intake can pose challenges for individuals with diabetes in managing blood glucose levels and weight. The generally high glycemic load of Western diet foods can deliver a substantial amount of rapidly digestible carbohydrates, straining the pancreas and inducing difficulties in managing diabetes by causing spikes and subsequent crashes in blood sugar levels.

The increased consumption of simple sugars, particularly high-fructose corn syrup, in the Western diet raises concerns due to its association with an elevated likelihood of insulin resistance and T2D. Sucrose, primarily found in fruits and vegetables, accounts for approximately 30-35% of carbohydrate intake. Lactose, the main sugar in milk and processed foods, contributes to around 10-15% of total carbohydrate calories. While fructose naturally occurs in fruits and vegetables, a significant portion is consumed in the form of high-fructose corn syrup, which has been associated with metabolic disturbances and adverse health effects.

Carbohydrate digestion initiates in the mouth, stomach, and small intestine, where specific enzymes break down starches and disaccharides into more easily absorbed simpler sugars. This process differentiates between 'good' and 'bad' sugars, where whole-food sources are broken down more gradually, supporting steady energy and blood sugar levels, whereas refined sugars are quickly absorbed, leading to spikes. However, certain carbohydrates referred to as 'resistant starch' and undigested sugars bypass this process and reach the colon. Research, such as experiments with resistant starch in pasta, shows that these carbohydrates undergo fermentation by gut bacteria, producing fatty acids that support gut health and can positively influence insulin response. Even cooking methods matter; for example, baking sweet potatoes increases their impact on blood sugar compared to boiling.

The type and preparation of carbohydrates consumed can influence this process. Raw or minimally processed foods often contain higher amounts of resistant starch compared to highly processed counterparts, providing greater fuel for beneficial gut bacteria.

Complex carbohydrates, found in foods like vegetables, fruits, whole grains, and legumes, have a longer molecular structure, making them slower to digest and thus providing a steady and sustainable energy source. They promote blood sugar stability, aid in weight management, and support overall health. In contrast, simple carbohydrates, which are found in fruits, honey, and sweets, can cause abrupt spikes in blood sugar levels, leading to potential weight gain and difficulties in controlling blood sugar.

The DiabeteBalance Diet draws inspiration from the principles of the Mediterranean diet, as well as the Glycemic Index (GI) and Glycemic Load (GL) framework. This diet recommends that approximately 45-65% of daily caloric intake should come from carbohydrates, with a focus on nutrient-dense, low-GI, and low-GL carbohydrate sources. Additionally, the diet emphasizes the consumption of MACs and high-fiber foods. Diets rich in MACs promote the growth of beneficial gut bacteria and facilitate the production of SCFAs, contributing to overall health improvements, including better blood sugar control.

Aligned with the 2020-2025 Dietary Guidelines, the DiabeteBalance Diet prioritizes the quality of carbohydrates rather than quantity. For effective weight loss and diabetes management, the diet encourages the consumption of foods with a low GI and GL, as well as a high fiber content. The DiabeteBalance Diet utilizes the GL of foods as a guiding principle, determining both the quality and quantity of carbohydrate consumption. This approach helps maintain stable blood sugar and insulin levels, aligning with the strategy outlined in the Twin Cycle Hypothesis for breaking the cycle of insulin resistance. By emphasizing high-quality carbohydrates—those that are low-GI, low-GL, and high in fiber—individuals have the potential to improve their metabolic health and reduce the likelihood of T2D.

UNDERSTANDING PROTEINS

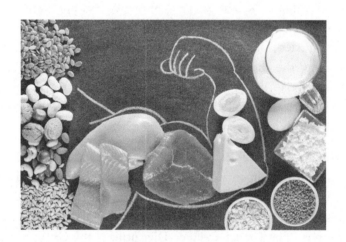

PROTEINS: ESSENTIAL FOR VITAL FUNCTIONS

Proteins are essential in various bodily functions, including tissue building and repair, hormone and enzyme production, fluid and acid-base balance, and immune function. They are the building blocks of life, contributing to the structural integrity of cells, organs, and tissues. From muscle fibers to enzymes that catalyze essential chemical reactions, proteins are involved in nearly every aspect of physiological processes.

PROTEIN IN THE WESTERN DIET

In the context of the Western diet, protein consumption often leans towards animal-based sources like meat, poultry, and dairy products. While these can provide complete sets of essential amino acids, the quality of proteins can vary. The Western diet frequently includes processed meats and high-fat cuts, which may not be the healthiest options. Emphasizing the quality of protein, such as choosing lean cuts, organic, or grass-fed sources, can make a significant difference in overall nutritional intake. The inclusion of plant-based proteins is often less pronounced but is gaining recognition for their health benefits and sustainability.

THE IMPORTANCE OF PROTEIN IN DIABETES MANAGEMENT

For individuals with insulin resistance or prediabetes, protein deficiency can worsen their condition and hinder the body's ability to effectively regulate glucose levels. Protein plays a crucial role in supporting insulin sensitivity, promoting the maintenance of healthy blood sugar levels. When protein intake is inadequate, the body may struggle to control glucose, leading to fluctuations in blood sugar and challenges in diabetes management. Convergent studies indicate that people with diabetes may have a protein deficiency ranging from 35 to 55%, according to various studies. This problem becomes even more severe in people with both diabetes and chronic kidney disease.

Addressing Protein Deficiency in Diabetes

Proteins are composed of a set of 20 standard amino acids, each with unique properties. These amino acids can form bonds with each other in various sequences, resulting in a diverse range of protein structures. This diversity is essential for the complex biological processes that sustain life. Among these amino acids, nine are considered essential because the body cannot produce them internally and they must be obtained through the diet. These essential amino acids play crucial roles in various physiological processes, including protein synthesis, growth, tissue repair, and maintenance. Additionally, they are involved in producing enzymes, hormones, and neurotransmitters, which are essential for proper bodily functioning.

According to the guidance of the American Diabetes Association (ADA), patients with diabetes and early stages of chronic kidney disease should aim for a protein intake of 0.8–1.0 g/kg per day, reducing it to 0.8 g/kg per day in the later stages of kidney disease. Adequate protein consumption is of utmost importance in enhancing the overall health and well-being of people with diabetes, as it helps prevent the decline of muscle mass and reduces the likelihood of falls and injuries.

Animal-based protein sources, including meat, poultry, fish, eggs, and dairy products, are widely recognized as complete protein sources. These sources typically contain all the essential amino acids required by the body. Plant-based proteins, found in legumes, grains, nuts, and seeds, may lack certain essential amino acids individually. However, incorporating a variety of plant-based proteins into the daily diet makes it possible to obtain all the essential amino acids required.

PROTEIN IN THE WESTERN DIET AND EMPHASIZING QUALITY

In the typical Western diet, protein often comes from meat, dairy products, and processed food sources. While these can provide essential amino acids, protein quality is often compromised by unhealthy fats, industrially made fats, and a mixture of oils commonly found in fast foods and convenience foods.

Particularly concerning is the Western diet's high ratio of omega-6 to omega-3 fatty acids, sometimes exceeding 15:1, compared to the recommended ratio of 4:1 or even lower. This imbalance, largely due to the consumption of certain vegetable oils, can lead to increased inflammation, insulin resistance, and other health risks.

COLLAGEN: THE UNDERESTIMATED PROTEIN

Collagen is one of the most prevalent proteins in the body. It is vital for preserving the integrity and elasticity of various tissues such as skin, hair, nails, bones, and joints. Its importance becomes more pronounced as we age, particularly after 50, as natural collagen production diminishes, leading to wrinkles, joint pain, and other aging symptoms. Collagen can be obtained through dietary sources such as bone broth, chicken skin, fish scales, and gelatin-rich meats. Additionally, collagen supplements have become popular for their convenience and effectiveness in providing this essential protein.

RED MEAT CONTROVERSY AND IMPORTANCE IN DIET

Red meats have been the subject of much debate and controversy, particularly in relation to heart health and cancer risks. While excessive consumption of processed and fatty cuts can contribute to these risks, red meat can still be part of a healthy diet when chosen wisely and consumed in moderation. Lean cuts like sirloin, tenderloin, and round steaks are lower in fat and provide essential nutrients like iron, vitamin B12, and zinc. Moreover, the way meat is cooked plays a significant role in its health impact. Methods such as grilling, roasting, or stewing that minimize added fats and carcinogenic compounds are generally recommended over frying or charbroiling.

COOKING METHODS AND PROTEIN QUALITY

The method used to cook protein sources can have a profound impact on their nutritional quality. Overcooking or using high-heat methods can denature proteins, reduce their digestibility, and lead to the formation of harmful compounds. Gentle cooking techniques like steaming, poaching, or slow cooking preserve the integrity of proteins and other essential nutrients. Marinating meats in antioxidant-rich ingredients like herbs, citrus, or vinegar can also help mitigate the formation of harmful substances during cooking.

PROTEIN IN YOUR DIET

Incorporating a well-balanced mix of protein sources into the diet can be advantageous for individuals with diabetes, helping to stabilize blood sugar levels, improve insulin sensitivity, and support overall health. A combination of lean animal-based proteins, collagen-rich sources, and plant-based options can provide the essential amino acids needed to maintain a healthy body and effectively manage diabetes. By recognizing the significance of protein in vital bodily functions and its role in diabetes management, individuals can make informed dietary choices to enhance their well-being and achieve better blood sugar control. Emphasizing quality, variety, and mindful cooking methods further aligns protein intake with broader health goals, promoting overall well-being and preventing the onset of chronic diseases.

FATS: ESSENTIAL MACRONUTRIENTS FOR OPTIMAL HEALTH

THE WESTERN DIET AND ULTRA-PROCESSED FATS

The Western Diet (WD), typified by its heavy reliance on processed foods, has become synonymous with the overconsumption of unhealthy fats. These fats often undergo ultra-processing techniques, which can strip away nutritional benefits and leave behind a mixture of oils riddled with trans fats and saturated fats. This is particularly noticeable in fast foods and convenience foods. The ultra-processing of fats, like the hydrogenation of vegetable oils, leads to industrially-made trans fats that have been linked to various health problems.

FATS: ESSENTIAL MACRONUTRIENTS FOR OPTIMAL HEALTH

Saturated Fats

Found mainly in animal products and specific plant-based sources like coconut oil, saturated fats have been controversial. Overconsumption can increase LDL ("bad") cholesterol levels, potentially contributing to heart disease and other cardiovascular issues. While essential in moderation, experts generally advise limiting saturated fat intake.

Unsaturated Fats

Considered healthier, unsaturated fats include monounsaturated and polyunsaturated fats. These fats can enhance blood cholesterol levels and improve heart health. Key sources include olive oil, avocados, nuts, fatty fish, seeds, and specific vegetable oils. However, it's essential to recognize that not all vegetable oils are beneficial. Some, like those high in omega-6 fatty acids, may create an imbalance in the omega-6 to omega-3 ratio, which can be inflammatory if not monitored.

Trans Fats

Created artificially through hydrogenation to solidify liquid oils, trans fats are a significant concern in processed and prepackaged foods. They can both raise LDL cholesterol and lower HDL ("good") cholesterol, causing substantial threats to heart health and overall well-being.

Misconception About Cholesterol

A widely held misconception is the excessive influence of dietary cholesterol on blood cholesterol levels. The liver naturally synthesizes a considerable amount of cholesterol, often far more than dietary intake. Recent research has shown that for most people, dietary cholesterol has a minimal effect on blood cholesterol levels, shifting the focus more towards the types of fats consumed rather than cholesterol itself.

UNHEALTHY FATS IN THE WESTERN DIET

The pervasive Western diet, characterized by an imbalanced intake of omega-6 fatty acids, saturated fats, trans fats, and deficiency in omega-3 fatty acids, can incite inflammation, insulin resistance, and Type 2 Diabetes (T2D). In some Western diets, the ratio of omega-6 to omega-3 has been found to be higher by as much as 20-fold from the recommended 4:1 or lower ratio. This imbalance has been linked to various health problems.

Olive Oil and the Mediterranean Diet

Olive oil, abundant in monounsaturated fats and antioxidants, is a cornerstone of the Mediterranean diet. Its consumption has been linked to a plethora of health advantages such as enhanced insulin responsiveness, diminished inflammation, and better heart health. Prioritizing olive oil over other less beneficial vegetable oils can be a vital step in managing diabetes and promoting overall well-being.

Recommended Intake and Effects on Diabetes Risk

Different types of fats have various effects on the risk for T2D. While dietary fat doesn't directly affect blood sugar levels, the quality of fats consumed can influence insulin sensitivity and T2D risk. High saturated fatty acids (SFAs) diets might increase T2D risk, whereas diets rich in polyunsaturated fatty acids (PUFAs) can confer protective effects.

Here are daily fat intake guidelines:

- **Saturated Fats:** Generally, less than 10% of total daily calories.
- **Unsaturated Fats:** These should be the majority of fat intake.
- **Trans Fats:** The World Health Organization advises a trans fat intake of less than 1% of total energy.

Adhering to these guidelines can boost insulin sensitivity and align with a balanced and nutrient-dense diet approach, emphasizing the importance of recognizing the complexity of fats in our diet.

UNDERSTANDING MICRONUTRIENTS

OVERVIEW OF NUTRIENTS: MICRONUTRIENTS AND MACRONUTRIENTS

Our bodies require various nutrients to function optimally. While macronutrients like fats, proteins, and carbohydrates provide the energy we need, micronutrients, although required in smaller quantities, are crucial for maintaining health, growth, and development. The deprivation of these vital nutrients can lead to severe deficiencies, causing pain and disease.

MICRONUTRIENTS

Micronutrients are classified into two main categories: vitamins and minerals. They are essential for several biological functions, such as energy production, immune function, bone health, and enzyme activation.

Vitamins: These are divided into fat-soluble (A, D, E, K) and water-soluble (B-vitamins, Vitamin C) groups. A deficiency in Vitamin D, for example, is linked to numerous diseases, including rickets in children and osteoporosis in adults, and has been correlated with increased risks of cancer, autoimmune disorders, and cardiovascular diseases.

Minerals: These include essential elements like calcium, magnesium, zinc, and iron, which are vital for various physiological functions.

THE WESTERN DIET AND MICRONUTRIENT DEFICIENCIES

The Western Diet (WD), characterized by a high intake of ultra-processed foods, often leads to imbalances and deficiencies in essential micronutrients. It can be rich in energy but poor in nutritional value, thus contributing to health issues like obesity, cardiovascular diseases, and metabolic syndrome, including Type 2 Diabetes (T2D). The overreliance on processed foods and lack of fresh, whole foods can lead to deficiencies in essential nutrients, such as Vitamin D, B-vitamins, and essential minerals.

THE DIABETEBALANCE DIET: AN INTEGRATED APPROACH

The DiabeteBalance Diet represents a meticulously crafted approach that recognizes the intricate interplay of nutrients. This diet focuses on both macronutrients and micronutrients, ensuring a balanced intake tailored to individual needs.

Harmonious Nutrient Pairs

The diet emphasizes nutrient pairs, such as Vitamin D and Calcium, which work synergistically to enhance nutrient absorption and bolster bone strength. Other essential pairings include Vitamin B12 and Folate, crucial for cell division and replication.

Managing Mineral Conflicts

Guidance on potential conflicts between minerals, like zinc and copper, ensures nutritional balance and helps avoid deficiencies or excesses that could lead to health problems.

Micronutrients in diabetes Management

Micronutrients play a significant role in managing diabetes by contributing to improved blood glucose regulation. The DiabeteBalance Diet focuses on:

- **Vitamin D:** Enhances insulin sensitivity.
- **Vitamin K:** Increases insulin sensitivity.
- **Magnesium:** Activates metabolic enzymes involved in glucose uptake.
- **Vitamin C:** Protects against oxidative stress.
- **B-Vitamins:** Vital for energy production and nerve function.
- **Chromium:** Regulates blood sugar levels.
- **Zinc:** Contributes to insulin sensitivity.
- **Calcium:** Works with Vitamin D for bone health and other functions.

By prioritizing and integrating the complex interplay of both macronutrients and micronutrients, the DiabeteBalance Diet offers a comprehensive, well-rounded strategy for managing diabetes. It also promotes overall well-being, highlighting the importance of nutrients that often go overlooked in the typical Western dietary pattern. The recognition of the vital role of micronutrients in human health can guide dietary choices towards better disease prevention, management, and optimal health.

UNDERSTANDING GUT HEALTH AND MICROBIOME

The gut microbiome is a complex ecosystem, housing trillions of microorganisms, predominantly bacteria, along with fungi and viruses, residing in our digestive system. These tiny inhabitants are pivotal to our well-being, influencing aspects ranging from metabolism to immune response. The connection between the gut microbiome and diabetes management is increasingly spotlighted in research.

Western Diet's Impact on Gut Health The Western Diet (WD) is marked by its significant consumption of processed foods, refined sugars, detrimental fats, and scarce fiber. Such a diet has been linked to disturbances in the gut microbiome, termed dysbiosis. This dietary pattern can skew the equilibrium between good and bad bacteria in the gut, paving the way for health complications, including insulin resistance and diabetes.

DYSBIOSIS AND ITS IMPACT

- **Metabolic Functions:** Dysbiosis can disrupt the fermentation of dietary fibers, resulting in a decline in the production of short-chain fatty acids (SCFAs). These SCFAs play a crucial role in regulating glucose metabolism and insulin sensitivity.

- **Inflammation:** Imbalances in the gut microbiome can cause chronic low-grade inflammation, contributing to insulin resistance.
- **Gut Barrier Function:** The compromised gut lining, commonly known as "leaky gut," can facilitate the leakage of toxins into the bloodstream, leading to inflammation and metabolic dysfunction.
- **Bile Acid Metabolism:** Changes in the gut microbiome can affect bile acid profiles, impacting metabolic health.

THE DIABETEBALANCE DIET: A FOCUS ON GUT HEALTH

Considering the role of gut health in diabetes, the DiabeteBalance Diet aims to nourish the gut microbiome through specific strategies:

High-fiber Diet

Emphasizing fiber-rich foods from diverse plant-based sources encourages the growth of beneficial bacteria, enhancing the production of SCFAs, and improving insulin sensitivity.

Probiotics and Prebiotics

Incorporating probiotics and prebiotics helps restore a healthy balance in the gut microbiome, fostering beneficial bacteria, and suppressing harmful ones.

Polyphenol-rich Foods

Consuming foods rich in polyphenols, like berries, green tea, and cocoa, not only offers antioxidant benefits but can also modulate the gut microbiome favorably.

Reduced Intake of Added Sugars and Highly Processed Foods

Minimizing the consumption of added sugars and ultra-processed foods supports a healthy gut microbiome by reducing the growth of harmful bacteria.

Integration of Healthy Fats

Including sources of healthy fats, like omega-3 fatty acids, can reduce inflammation and support a more balanced gut environment.

***

THE DIABETEBALANCE DIET AS A COMPREHENSIVE APPROACH

The DiabeteBalance Diet represents an innovative and integrated approach to managing diabetes by focusing on the gut microbiome. By recognizing the intricate connection between dietary patterns, gut health, and metabolic functions, this diet offers a pathway to improve not only diabetes management but overall well-being. By moving away from the typical Western Diet pattern and embracing whole, nutrient-dense foods, individuals can promote a healthier gut microbiome, enhance insulin sensitivity, and take proactive steps towards a healthier life.

PART III
UNDERSTANDING
DIABETEBALANCE DIET

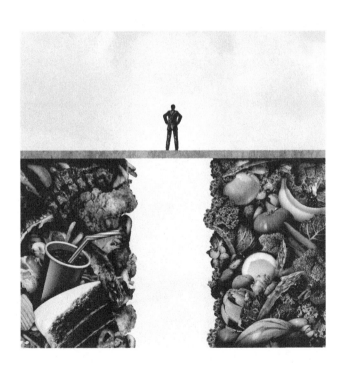

THE DIABETEBALANCE DIET: INTRODUCTION

In today's ever-evolving world of nutritional science, effectively managing diabetes remains a critical challenge in healthcare. As the prevalence of diabetes continues to grow worldwide, the demand for a sustainable and efficient dietary strategy becomes increasingly urgent. The DiabeteBalance Diet rises to meet this need by incorporating the core principles of the Mediterranean Diet, Glycemic Index, and Glycemic Load to create a comprehensive approach to diabetes management and weight loss.

The Mediterranean Diet, renowned for its association with heart health, longevity, and overall well-being, forms a foundational pillar of the DiabeteBalance Diet. Emphasizing whole foods, healthy fats, lean proteins, and a diverse range of fruits and vegetables, this dietary framework introduces essential elements that align perfectly with the goals of optimal health and diabetes management.

Complementing the Mediterranean Diet, the Glycemic Index (GI) and Glycemic Load (GL) contribute to a nuanced understanding of blood sugar regulation. The GI measures how different foods impact blood glucose levels, while the GL provides a more precise insight by considering both the GI and the quantity consumed. These principles enable precise control over dietary factors that influence blood sugar, offering a targeted approach to managing diabetes.

What sets the DiabeteBalance Diet apart is its integration of these diverse dietary principles into a unified, cohesive plan. This integrated approach surpasses traditional dietary guidelines, providing a multifaceted strategy not only for controlling blood glucose levels but also for enhancing insulin sensitivity, promoting weight loss, and improving overall metabolic health.

In the following chapters, we will delve into each of these concepts in detail, elucidating their individual roles within the DiabeteBalance Diet and how they synergistically promote health and well-being. By exploring the Mediterranean Diet, Glycemic Index, and Glycemic Load, you will gain a comprehensive understanding of the underlying principles that define the DiabeteBalance Diet. Armed with this knowledge, you will be equipped with a solid foundation to adopt a more informed and strategic approach to managing diabetes, grounded in both time-tested dietary wisdom and contemporary nutritional insights.

THE DIABETEBALANCE DIET
FRAMEWORK: BUILDING BLOCKS
FOR SUCCESS

THE DIABETEBALANCE DIET FRAMEWORK: BUILDING BLOCKS FOR SUCCESS

The DiabeteBalance Diet represents a meticulous and comprehensive approach to managing diabetes and enhancing overall well-being. Integrating the foundational principles of the Mediterranean Diet with the discerning insights of the Glycemic Index (GI) and Glycemic Load (GL), this synergistic fusion not only targets blood glucose regulation but also crafts strategies for weight management, cardiovascular health, and metabolic function optimization.

THE MEDITERRANEAN DIET

The DiabeteBalance Diet's first cornerstone is the time-honored Mediterranean Diet, celebrated for its profound cardiovascular benefits and life-extending qualities. This dietary paradigm thrives on the consumption of a varied spectrum of nutrient-dense foods, emphasizing fruits, vegetables, whole grains, legumes, wholesome fats like olive oil, and lean proteins, especially fish. By adopting the Mediterranean Diet, the DiabeteBalance Diet sets the stage for a nourishing, palatable, and enduring dietary regimen that aligns perfectly with the objectives of diabetes control.

THE GLYCEMIC INDEX AND GLYCEMIC LOAD

The second cornerstone of the DiabeteBalance Diet involves the integration of the principles of the Glycemic Index and Glycemic Load. The GI serves as a valuable ranking tool, categorizing foods based on their impact on blood glucose levels, empowering individuals with diabetes to make informed and intelligent dietary choices. The GL further fine-tunes this methodology by considering both the GI value and the portion size of the food. This dual consideration enables the DiabeteBalance Diet to exert more refined control over blood sugar levels, a crucial aspect of successful diabetes management.

ALIGNING WITH INDIVIDUAL NEEDS

Recognizing the diversity of needs and preferences among individuals, the DiabeteBalance Diet embraces the significance of personalized nutrition. By allowing the customization of dietary selections within the established framework, it ensures congruence with unique health aspirations and lifestyle considerations. This tailored adaptability lies at the heart of the diet's efficacy, promoting a sustainable and practical approach that resonates with daily life.

FOSTERING SYNERGY FOR HOLISTIC WELLNESS

The components of the DiabeteBalance Diet work together harmoniously rather than in isolation. In addition to diet, the diet recognizes the vital role of ancillary factors such as consistent physical activity, sufficient sleep, and adept stress management. By acknowledging that well-being is multi-dimensional, the DiabeteBalance Diet champions a holistic lifestyle regimen that amplifies each person's ability to manage disease and elevate overall health.

In summation, the DiabeteBalance Diet Framework provides a comprehensive path to managing diabetes and promoting holistic health. By incorporating the principles of the Mediterranean Diet, the Glycemic Index, and Glycemic Load, this diet offers a unified and scientifically supported approach to nutrition. As readers delve into each foundational element in the following chapters, they will discover a structured blueprint for achieving success in diabetes management and enhancing overall well-being.

THE MEDITERRANEAN DIET EXPLAINED: A PATHWAY TO HEALTH AND WELL-BEING

The Mediterranean diet is not merely a meal plan; it embodies a rich cultural tradition and a holistic approach to nourishing the body and soul. Inspired by the time-honored eating habits of countries bordering the Mediterranean Sea, this dietary pattern has captured the world's attention due to its numerous health benefits and recognition as one of the healthiest diets globally. Characterized by an abundance of fresh fruits, raw vegetables, whole grains, olive oil, nuts, seeds, and lean proteins, the Mediterranean diet is more than just a trend—it is a way of life that has stood the test of time.

The origins of the Mediterranean diet can be traced back to the early 1960s, when researchers noticed that individuals living in the Mediterranean region had reduced rates of chronic diseases, such as heart disease and cancer. This observation led to the groundbreaking Seven Countries Study, conducted by the esteemed nutritionist Ancel Keys, which shed light on the potential health benefits of the Mediterranean diet. Since then, an ever-expanding body of scientific research has consistently supported its positive impact on health, making it a favored option for those striving to enhance their overall well-being and longevity.

The heart of the Mediterranean diet lies not just in its carefully selected ingredients but in the way it fosters a harmonious relationship between food, family, and community. Mealtime in Mediterranean cultures is a cherished affair, where shared dishes and leisurely dining are central to the experience. This cultural aspect of the diet reinforces the notion that food is more than just sustenance—it is a celebration of life, love, and togetherness.

KEY COMPONENTS OF THE MEDITERRANEAN DIET: BUILDING A NUTRIENT-RICH PLATE

Abundance of Plant-Based Foods: The Foundation of Vitality

At the heart of the Mediterranean diet lies an abundance of plant-based foods, providing a treasure trove of essential nutrients. Fruits and vegetables take center stage, offering a vibrant array of colors, flavors, and health benefits. Rich in vitamins, minerals, antioxidants, and dietary fiber, these plant-based powerhouses nourish the body and support overall health.

Whole grains, like barley, bulgur, quinoa, such as barley, bulgur, quinoa, and a variety of others, add depth and substance to meals while providing slow-digesting carbohydrates that sustain energy levels and promote stable blood sugar. The Mediterranean diet's focus on whole grains ensures that each bite is not just delicious but also wholesome, supporting digestive health and overall well-being.

Olive Oil: The Golden Elixir of Health

Olive oil, cherished as the "liquid gold" of the Mediterranean, serves as the primary source of fat in this diet. Renowned for its rich, fruity flavor and health-promoting properties, extra virgin olive oil is a treasure trove of monounsaturated fats, particularly oleic acid. These heart-healthy fats help lower LDL cholesterol levels, reducing the likelihood of heart disease while promoting the elevation of HDL cholesterol, the "good" cholesterol.

Moreover, extra virgin olive oil boasts an impressive array of antioxidants and polyphenols, such as vitamin E and hydroxytyrosol, which defend the body against oxidative stress and inflammation. This golden elixir not only adds a delectable touch to dishes but also bestows a host of health benefits.

Balancing Fish and Poultry: A Bounty of Protein

The Mediterranean diet embraces a moderate consumption of fish and poultry, offering an abundance of lean protein sources. Fatty fish, including salmon, sardines, and mackerel, present an omega-3 fatty acid treasure trove, particularly EPA and DHA. These essential fatty acids are crucial for heart health, brain function, and inflammation reduction, providing a powerful defense against chronic diseases.

Poultry, such as chicken and turkey, adds to the protein bounty of the Mediterranean diet, supporting muscle repair, immune function, and overall cellular health.

Limiting Red Meat and Sweets: A Harmony of Moderation

While the Mediterranean diet acknowledges the appeal of red meat, it encourages its consumption in moderation. When indulging in red meat, the focus is on lean cuts and smaller portion sizes to maintain balance and reduce the risk of certain health conditions.

Sweets and processed foods are treated as occasional treats in the Mediterranean diet. Instead, the diet celebrates the natural sweetness of fruits, offering a nourishing alternative to sugary temptations.

HEALTH BENEFITS OF THE MEDITERRANEAN DIET: A SYMPHONY OF WELLNESS

The Mediterranean diet is celebrated for its profound impact on overall health and well-being. Its health benefits have been extensively studied and include:

Cardiovascular Health

Various studies have demonstrated that adhering to MedDiet can significantly lessen the likelihood of cardiovascular diseases. The abundance of heart-healthy monounsaturated fats in olive oil and omega-3 fatty acids in fish, along with a diet abundant in antioxidants and anti-inflammatory compounds, contributes to improved blood pressure, cholesterol levels, and overall heart function.

A 2013-study published in "The New England Journal of Medicine" revealed that individuals who adhered to the MedDiet rich in extra virgin olive oil or nuts experienced a remarkable 30% reduction in the risk of strokes, heart attacks, and other cardiovascular-related mortality when compared to those following a low-fat diet.

Diabetes Management and Prevention

The Mediterranean diet has shown promise in managing and preventing type 2 diabetes. Its low-glycemic index and emphasis on whole foods contribute to better blood sugar control, reduced insulin resistance, and weight management. Moreover, the diet's focus on healthy fats helps maintain insulin sensitivity and can reduce the risk of developing diabetes.

A 2011-review published in the "American Journal of Clinical Nutrition" concluded that following the Mediterranean diet was linked to a reduced probability of developing type 2 diabetes.

Weight Loss and Weight Management

Though not primarily marketed as a weight loss diet, the Mediterranean diet can be effective for weight management. Its emphasis on nutrient-dense, filling foods like fruits, vegetables, and whole grains helps individuals feel satisfied and less likely to overeat. Moreover, the inclusion of healthy fats in the diet can help control appetite and provide sustained energy levels.

Several studies have supported the Mediterranean diet's positive impact on weight loss and maintenance. A randomized trial published in 2016 in the "Lancet Diabetes & Endocrinology" found that participants assigned to a Mediterranean diet with no caloric restriction lost more weight than those on a low-fat diet with calorie restriction.

Brain Health

Studies have linked the Mediterranean diet to enhanced cognitive function and a reduced likelihood of developing neurodegenerative diseases, such as Alzheimer's. The diet's high intake of antioxidants and anti-inflammatory compounds, along with the presence of healthy fats, may contribute to these benefits.

A 2015-study published in "JAMA Internal Medicine" showed that adherence to MedDiet was linked to slower cognitive degeneration and a lowered risk of Alzheimer's disease.

Cancer Prevention

The Mediterranean diet's focus on whole, minimally plant-based foods, phenol-rich foods, and healthy fats has been associated with a lessened risk of certain types of cancer, particularly breast and colorectal cancers. The antioxidants and phytochemicals found in fruits, vegetables, and olive oil help preserve cells from damage and lessen the probability of cancer development.

A 2019-review published in "Nutrients" found that close adherence to the MedDiet was associated with a reduced risk of breast cancer.

Practical Tips for Adopting the Mediterranean Diet

Adopting the MedDiet can be a tasty and enjoyable experience. Here are some practical tips to help you embark on this gastronomic adventure:

- Incorporate More Fruits and Vegetables: Aim to fill half your plate with a variety of colorful fruits and vegetables in every meal. Snack on veggies and/or fruits between meals for added nutrition and vitality.
- Choose Whole Grains: Opt for whole grains like barley, quinoa, and bulgur instead of refined grains. Use whole-grain bread and pasta in your meals to maximize their health benefits.
- Use Olive Oil: Replace unhealthy fats with olive oil or EVOO for cooking and salad dressings. Drizzle olive oil on vegetables and use it as a dip for whole-grain bread to savor its rich flavors and nutritional prowess.
- Eat Fish and Poultry: Include fatty fish and lean poultry in your diet a few times a week for a good source of protein. Bake or grill them with herbs and spices for added flavor and health benefits.
- Limit Red Meat and Sweets: Reduce the consumption of red meat and sweets to occasional treats. Instead, choose plant-based proteins like legumes and nuts for your meals to maintain balance and overall well-being.
- Stay Hydrated: Drink plenty of water throughout the day and limit sugary beverages. Herbal teas and infused water can be refreshing alternatives that hydrate your body and invigorate your senses.
- Enjoy Meals Mindfully: Savor your meals, eat slowly, and enjoy the social aspect of dining with family and friends. Avoid distractions like television or electronic devices during mealtime to fully immerse in the pleasure of eating.
- Cook at Home: Embrace the art of cooking and prepare homemade meals whenever possible. Cooking at home allows you to have full control over the ingredients and cooking

methods, enabling you to savor the tastes and nourishment of each dish.

The Mediterranean diet is not just a fleeting trend or a rigid set of rules—it is a symphony of tastes, nourishment, and cultural heritage that nurtures both the body and soul. By embracing this wholesome and sustainable way of eating, individuals can enhance their overall well-being and cultivate a lifelong journey of good health.

The MedDiet is more than just a diet; it is a pathway to optimal health and longevity. Its benefits extend beyond physical health to encompass mental well-being and a sense of connection to culture and tradition. It reminds us that food is not merely a means of sustenance but a vital source of nourishment.

GLYCEMIC LOAD: THE MISSING LINK IN DIABETES MANAGEMENT

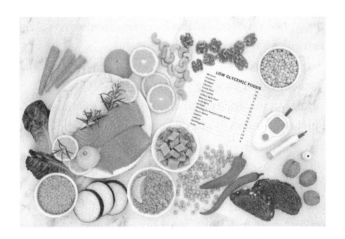

Managing Type 2 diabetes effectively requires a thorough comprehension of the scientific principles that shape our dietary choices. To design the DiabeteBalance Diet, which aims to address all key facets of a diabetes-management and health-promoting diet, the MECE (Mutually Exclusive, Collectively Exhaustive) framework has been applied. This framework ensures that every diet component serves a unique function (mutually exclusive) and includes all the essentials for a comprehensive and balanced diet (collectively exhaustive). By satisfying these conditions, the DiabeteBalance Diet becomes a holistic and potent dietary strategy for optimally managing diabetes and promoting effective weight management.

UNDERSTANDING THE GLYCEMIC INDEX AND GLYCEMIC LOAD

The DiabeteBalance Diet places significant emphasis on the principles of Glycemic Index (GI) and Glycemic Load (GL). The Glycemic Index was introduced by Dr. David Jenkins and his team at the University of Toronto in 1981 to enhance our understanding of how carbohydrate-rich foods impact blood glucose levels. It assigns a numerical score to foods, indicating their relative speed in raising blood sugar compared to a reference food. Based on their scores, foods are categorized as low, medium, or high glycemic index:

- Low glycemic index foods: GI less than 55
- Medium glycemic index foods: GI between 56 and 69
- High glycemic index foods: GI more than 70

The initial focus of the Glycemic Index (GI) was to encourage the consumption of low-GI foods, moderate intake of medium-GI foods, and avoidance of high-GI foods. However, this approach had a notable limitation as it did not consider portion sizes. It is important to note that consuming large quantities of low-GI foods, such as skim milk with a relatively high sugar content per serving (24.9g of total sugars per 16 oz), could still result in elevated blood glucose levels. Moreover, solely emphasizing the GI may lead to the consumption of potentially unhealthy low-GI foods and overlook the significance of a balanced diet.

Refining the Glycemic Index with Glycemic Load

To overcome the limitations of the GI, Harvard University

researchers introduced the concept of Glycemic Load (GL). The GL considers both the carbohydrates' quality and quantity in a specific food portion, providing a more holistic measure of its influence on blood sugar levels. Foods are categorized into low, medium, and high glycemic load based on their GL values. The DiabeteBalance Diet considers both the Glycemic Index and the Glycemic Load when assessing the impact of food on blood sugar levels. This approach emphasizes carbohydrate quality, portion control, and calorie consciousness. In the GL system, 1 GL unit signifies the effect of consuming 1 gram of pure glucose.

Foods are categorized based on their Glycemic Load:

- Low GL: 10 or less
- Medium GL: 11 to 19
- High GL: 20 or more

The Glycemic Load (GL) plays a pivotal role in the DiabeteBalance Diet. It considers both the Glycemic Index and the quantity of carbohydrates consumed in a single serving when assessing its effect on blood sugar levels. This approach, besides emphasizing carbohydrate quality, underscores the importance of portion control and calorie consciousness.

For instance, while watermelon has a high Glycemic Index (GI), its overall Glycemic Load is low due to the modest amount of carbohydrates in a serving. A serving of watermelon, roughly 1 cup (152g), only contains 11 grams of carbohydrates, resulting in a lower Glycemic Load despite a high GI.

Conversely, despite being a low-GI food, parsnips have a higher carbohydrate content. A cooked parsnip serving about 1 cup (215g) contains 35 grams of carbohydrates. This relatively high carbohydrate content results in a higher Glycemic Load compared to watermelon, despite watermelon's higher GI.

THE TWIN CYCLE HYPOTHESIS AND ITS IMPACT ON MANAGING T2D THROUGH FAT ACCUMULATION CONTROL

The Twin Cycle Hypothesis, proposed by Prof. Roy Taylor and his team at Newcastle University, UK, offers valuable insights into the development and treatment of T2D. According to this hypothesis, the disease is initiated by two interconnected cycles: the accumulation of fat in the liver and the accumulation of fat in the pancreas.

The first cycle primarily involves the liver. When individuals consume an excessive amount of calories that surpass their body's needs, the surplus energy is stored as fat in the liver. This buildup of fat hampers the liver's ability to respond to insulin, leading to heightened blood sugar levels. In order to counteract insulin resistance, the pancreas increases its insulin production as a compensatory mechanism.

The second cycle involves the pancreas. The heightened production of insulin contributes to the buildup of fat in the pancreas, which adversely affects the function of beta cells responsible for insulin production. As the function of beta cells deteriorates, insulin resistance worsens, establishing a destructive cycle that ultimately leads to the development of T2D.

Understanding the Twin Cycle Hypothesis has significant implications for the treatment of T2D. If the accumulation of fat in the liver and pancreas is the underlying cause, then reversing this fat accumulation could ultimately reverse the condition itself. Research has indicated that implementing a diet restricted in calories has demonstrated the ability to reduce fat accumulation in both the liver and pancreas. This fat content reduction contributes to restoring normal insulin production and function.

This insight represents a significant shift in the approach to managing T2D. Instead of solely concentrating on symptom control, the focus is now on tackling the underlying cause of the disease. By specifically addressing the accumulation of fat in the liver and pancreas, it opens up the potential to develop highly effective strategies for both preventing and optimally managing diabetes.

CARB COUNTING AND THE GLYCEMIC LOAD

New studies suggest that the amount of carbs in a meal has a less significant impact on your blood glucose and insulin changes than the glycemic load. The GL is a more accurate predictor of post-meal blood sugar and insulin response compared to simply counting carbs.

Carb Counting Guidelines for Diabetes

Previously, it was believed that both the amount and type of carbohydrates in food would determine blood sugar levels. For instance, eating fifty grams of pure sugar was assumed to cause the same blood glucose response as any fifty-gram carbohydrate-containing food. However, this idea is now proven to be incorrect.

Carbohydrates in the food you consume will elevate your blood glucose levels. The rate at which this occurs depends on the quality of the carbs and what you consume them with. For example, the sugar levels in fruit or vegetable juice cause a notable spike in blood sugar levels, whereas sugar in whole fruits or vegetables is digested more slowly. Carbohydrate-containing foods will be digested slower if consumed with fat, fiber, or protein, leading to gentler increases in blood sugar levels.

Carb counting, or tracking the carbohydrates in all your meals, snacks, and drinks, is an essential tool for those with diabetes. This practice can help manage blood sugar levels, which in turn can:

- Avoid dramatic spikes in blood sugar levels

- Prolong overall health and reduce the severity of some diabetes complications
- Enhance the quality of life
- Prevent further diabetes complications such as eye disorders, kidney disease, foot ulcers, heart disease, and stroke

If you use mealtime or fast-acting insulin, you'll need to count carbohydrates to align your insulin dose with your carb intake.

Types of Carbohydrates in Your Diet

Upon consuming carbohydrates, your body breaks them down into glucose, which is then absorbed into the bloodstream. Dietary carbohydrates can be categorized into two groups:

- **Complex carbohydrates**, found in vegetables, fruits, peas, beans, and whole grains.
- **Simple carbohydrates** found in processed foods and refined sugars.

Choosing the Best Carbohydrate-Containing Foods

Frequently eating low-quality carbs (high glycemic foods) can lead to frequent blood sugar spikes, complicating blood sugar level control and causing inflammation, weight gain, obesity, insulin resistance, and cortisol dysregulation. On the other hand, fibers in whole foods (low glycemic foods) are known to mitigate these effects.

CARBOHYDRATE INTAKE IN DIABETES MANAGEMENT

The appropriate carbohydrate intake for optimal blood sugar control can vary significantly among individuals. Factors influencing this variation include age, gender, activity level, medication regimen, and overall health.

A common guideline, often endorsed by organizations like the American Diabetes Association, suggests that people with diabetes might aim for carbohydrates to constitute around 45% of their daily caloric intake. However, individual needs can diverge from this general recommendation.

Breakdown and Calculation:

To understand this in concrete terms, let's break down a 1,900-calorie diet:

If 45% of a 1,900-calorie diet should come from carbohydrates:

$45/100 \times 1,900 = 855$ calories are allotted for carbohydrates

Given that each gram of carbohydrate equates to 4 calories:

855 calories ÷ 4 calories/gram = 213.75 grams of carbs.

Thus, someone consuming a 1,900-calorie diet and following the 45% guideline would aim to incorporate approximately 214 grams of carbohydrates into their daily intake.

It's imperative for individuals with diabetes to collaborate with a their healthcare providers. Personalizing carbohydrate intake based on unique factors and regular blood sugar monitoring can optimize diabetes management. Some might find that their needs are better met with a higher or lower carbohydrate percentage, depending on their specific circumstances.

How Much GL Should I Aim for Each Day?

Low-glycemic diets can vary significantly, with many sources recommending daily Glycemic Load (GL) values between 80 to 150. For those aiming to maximize health benefits, targeting a daily GL under 100 could be advantageous. However, individuals with diabetes should consult with a healthcare professional to ascertain an appropriate daily GL, as individual requirements may vary. As a general guideline, it is essential not to exceed a daily GL of 50.

Carb Counting or Glycemic Load: Which is More Effective for Diabetes Management?

Carbohydrate counting remains a foundational tool in diabetes management, offering clarity on carbohydrate intake and its potential impact on blood sugar. However, the glycemic load introduces an added dimension, accounting for the quality of carbohydrates consumed. This can provide deeper insights into how foods might affect glucose levels. For a comprehensive approach, combining both carbohydrate counting and considering GL can be beneficial, granting a richer perspective for better diabetes control. Always collaborate with healthcare professionals when making dietary adjustments related to diabetes management.

High Insulin Levels and the Benefits of a Low-Glycemic Load Diet

High insulin levels, prompted by high glycemic index foods, are detrimental and may promote chronic issues such as elevated blood fat, high blood glucose, hypertension, and a heightened risk of heart attack. Consequently, following the glycemic load diet is advantageous in managing diabetes, preventing its complications, supporting weight loss in the mid and long-term and enhancing overall health.

Unlike trendy low-carbohydrate, high-protein diets, a low Glycemic Load diet has been scientifically validated to aid individuals in various ways, as explored in this chapter:

- Control blood sugar and insulin release
- Achieve and maintain a healthy weight
- Reduce Polycystic Ovary Syndrome (PCOS) symptoms
- Maintain a healthy condition
- Minimize the risk of type 2 diabetes
- Improve gestational diabetes management and mitigate adverse pregnancy outcomes

- Substantially decrease the risk of developing metabolic syndrome
- Prevent heart attacks and strokes

Low-Glycemic Load Diet and Insulin Resistance Reversal

Insulin resistance is a grave and covert health condition that develops when cells in the muscles, liver, and fat tissues begin to disregard the signal sent by the insulin hormone to transfer sugar from the bloodstream into body cells. As the condition develops, the body responds by continually producing more insulin to lower blood sugar.

Over time, the pancreas's β cells, strained by the need to generate an excessive supply of insulin, falter, and blood sugar levels rise, signaling pre-diabetes or, in the worst case, type 2 diabetes.

Insulin resistance remains undetected in its early stages and only manifests symptoms later when the pancreas can no longer release enough insulin to keep blood glucose within the normal range. These symptoms may include metabolic syndrome, polycystic ovary syndrome (PCOS), and various types of diabetes.

Fortunately, the deleterious effects of insulin resistance can be mitigated, and insulin sensitivity can be boosted by following a low-glycemic index diet. Such a diet is beneficial for managing health conditions sensitive to insulin resistance, such as:

- Excessive hunger
- Lethargy or fatigue
- Difficulty concentrating
- Brain fog
- Waist weight gain
- High blood pressure

LOW-GLYCEMIC LOAD DIET: A HEALTHIER OPTION

Natural foods like legumes, fruits, vegetables, meats, fish, and grains usually contain more complex carbohydrates, translating to a low-glycemic index. Consuming these foods leads to gradual increases and decreases in blood glucose levels, helping maintain a healthy condition, promoting weight loss, preventing obesity, and aiding in diabetes control.

Numerous studies have showcased the health advantages of low-glycemic index foods, including:

- Diabetes management (gestational, type 1, and type 2)
- Long-lasting weight loss
- Obesity control
- Reduction of heart strokes
- Prevention of coronary heart disease
- PCOS prevention

Low-Glycemic Diet and Hunger Reduction

Leptin, the "hunger hormone," is produced by fat tissues and plays a vital role in weight regulation by suppressing appetite.

Eating low-glycemic-index foods lowers the insulin response and increases circulating leptin levels, leading to reduced food consumption. This is highly beneficial for:

- Type 2 diabetes management
- Obesity control
- Weight loss
- Weight maintenance management
- Insulin resistance

When consuming a balanced combination of foods, appetite is controlled due to the leptin effect, insulin levels stabilize, and sugar levels rise and fall smoothly. These benefits lead to weight loss and support a healthy lifestyle.

INTEGRATING DIETARY STRATEGIES FOR EFFECTIVE DIABETES MANAGEMENT

Aligned with the Twin Cycle Hypothesis, the DiabeteBalance Diet combines the principles of the Glycemic Index, Glycemic Load, and the Mediterranean Diet. By integrating these dietary strategies, we can effectively target fat accumulation in the liver and pancreas, recognized as a pivotal factor in the onset of T2D.

The DiabeteBalance Diet emphasizes foods with a low Glycemic Load to prevent abrupt blood sugar and insulin surges, thus curbing fat deposition in the liver and pancreas. It also incorporates the nutrient-rich and anti-inflammatory properties of the Mediterranean Diet, which has been associated with enhanced insulin sensitivity and a decreased likelihood of developing T2D.

By merging the principles of the Glycemic Load diet and the Mediterranean Diet, the DiabeteBalance Diet becomes an effective dietary strategy for naturally managing Diabetes and potentially reversing T2D. This holistic and root cause-focused approach can potentially address this widespread metabolic disorder on a global scale, representing a critical shift in our strategies for managing T2D and paving the way for proactive and effective diabetes management.

KEY PRINCIPLES AND EVIDENCE OF THE DIABETEBALANCE DIET

The principles of the DiabeteBalance Diet are designed to be practical, adaptable, and sustainable, aligning seamlessly with other established healthy dietary patterns, such as the Mediterranean Diet and the recommendations of the 2020-2025 Dietary Guidelines for Americans. This integration enhances their effectiveness in optimally managing diabetes.

Understanding that the DiabeteBalance Diet is not merely a temporary solution but a lifelong commitment is essential. This approach aims to prevent fat re-accumulation in the liver and pancreas, consistent with the Twin Cycle Hypothesis for people with T2D. Reversal of T2D is marked by a sustained reduction in HbA1c levels to below 6.5% for at least three months, whether spontaneously or with intervention, and without the reliance on regular glucose-lowering medications.

To fully reap the rewards of the DiabeteBalance Diet, one must grasp and consistently apply its principles. While it may not require an all-or-nothing adherence initially, consistent application will yield substantial benefits, accelerating the optimal management of T2D.

These principles also extend beyond diabetes control, enhancing overall health and well-being.

Here are the 14 key principles of the DiabeteBalance Diet:

1. Embrace Low-Glycemic Load Foods: Choosing foods with a low glycemic load (GL) ensures that both the quality and amount of carbs ingested are controlled. Every unit of GL corresponds to 1 gram of pure glucose, which can raise awareness about dietary choices and portion control. Foods low in GL generally release glucose slowly and steadily, preventing sudden spikes in blood sugar levels.
2. Embrace a Mediterranean-Inspired Diet: The Mediterranean Diet, which emphasizes fruits, vegetables, whole grains, lean proteins, and healthy fats, provides an excellent dietary model for managing diabetes. By coupling this diet with a focus on GL, you can suppress unhealthy choices such as refined grains and sugary beverages, promoting a balanced, heart-healthy eating pattern.
3. Emphasize Nutrient Density: Prioritize foods abundant in essential nutrients (e.g., vitamins, minerals) but low in empty calories. Highly processed foods often lack nutritional value, offering calories without essential vitamins and minerals. Instead, opt for whole, unprocessed foods that support overall health and weight management.
4. Limit Intake of Added Sugars and Sweets: Limit drastically the consumption of foods high in added sugars and sweets to control blood glucose levels. Be aware of hidden added sugars found in processed foods and beverages; always check labels to make informed choices.
5. Reduce Consumption of Saturated Fats and Eliminate Trans Fats: Saturated fats should contribute only 5% to 6% of total calorie intake. Reducing these unhealthy fats and eliminating trans fats can enhance heart health and insulin sensitivity.
6. Choose Healthy Fats and Focus on Heart-Healthy Fats:

Include foods rich in monounsaturated and polyunsaturated fats, like avocados, nuts, seeds, and olive oil. Aim for an (omega-6 to omega-3 fatty acids) ratio of 4-5, incorporating omega-3-rich foods like fatty fish, flaxseeds, and walnuts to improve insulin sensitivity and reduce inflammation.

7. Pay Attention to Gut Health: Consuming fiber-rich foods supports a healthy gut microbiome, beneficial for diabetes management. A balanced gut can improve insulin sensitivity and strengthen the immune system, lowering the likelihood of inflammation and related health issues.

8. Include Anti-Inflammatory and Antioxidant Foods: Inflammation is linked to the onset and worsening of chronic illnesses. Include foods rich in anti-inflammatory and antioxidant compounds, like fruits, vegetables, and nuts, to combat oxidative stress and underlying inflammation.

9. Include Glucagon-Like Peptide Agonist Compounds: Foods like legumes and olive oil, rich in these compounds, help regulate blood sugar levels. Other sources include certain whole grains and dairy products.

10. Keep Balanced and Consistent Protein Intake: Focus on lean protein sources to maintain muscle mass and promote fullness. Follow Recommended Dietary Allowances (RDAs), targeting around 0.8 grams of protein per kilogram of body weight.

11. Stay Hydrated: Proper hydration is essential for regulating blood sugar. If you don't drink enough water, the glucose in your bloodstream becomes more concentrated, leading to higher blood sugar levels. Both mild and severe dehydration can significantly impact diabetes management.

12. Adopt and Sustain a Regular Physical Activity Routine: Regular exercise supports weight management and promotes cardiovascular health. For those with disabilities or weaknesses, low-impact exercises and activities guided by healthcare professionals can still provide significant benefits.

13. Emphasize Dietary Patterns: Focusing on overall dietary

patterns rather than isolated nutrients ensures a variety of nutrient-rich foods, offering a balanced and wholesome approach to eating.

14. Regular Health Check-Ups: Regular health monitoring helps in tracking progress and making necessary adjustments, collaborating with healthcare providers to ensure that individualized needs are met.

By incorporating these principles, those with diabetes or at risk can proactively manage their condition, boost overall wellness, and potentially ward off further complications. Structuring a diet and lifestyle around these guidelines forms a comprehensive and holistic strategy for thriving with diabetes.

Extensive scientific research and clinical trials have illuminated the effectiveness of the DiabeteBalance Diet in managing diabetes. These studies encompass various aspects such as Glycemic Index (GI), Glycemic Load (GL), the Mediterranean Diet, and the Twin Cycle Hypothesis, contributing to a robust understanding of this dietary approach's benefits.

Numerous studies underscore the positive influence of low-GI and low-GL diets on blood sugar regulation in T2D individuals. A comprehensive 2019-review in the "American Journal of Clinical Nutrition" affirmed that low-GI diets could significantly lower HbA1c levels compared to high-GI diets, reducing the risk of diabetes-related complications.

The Mediterranean Diet, integral to the DiabeteBalance Diet, has also demonstrated efficacy in T2D management. The landmark PRED-IMED study found that adherence to MedDiet, rich with extra-virgin olive oil or nuts, led to an remarkable 52% reduction in T2D development risk compared to a low-fat control diet.

The Twin Cycle Hypothesis, by Professor Roy Taylor, serves as the core of the DiabeteBalance Diet. This theory posits that T2D results from abnormal fat accumulation in the liver and pancreas. Professor Taylor's seminal research, including a major study in "The Lancet Diabetes & Endocrinology" in 2016, showed that a low-calorie diet causing significant weight loss could effectively reverse T2D by reducing fat levels in these organs.

Informed by the Twin Cycle Hypothesis, the DiabeteBalance Diet emphasizes weight loss and fat reduction in the liver and pancreas, and aligns with principles like low-GI, low-GL, and the Dietary Guidelines for Americans. It fosters nutrient-rich, calorie-conscious eating to lessen chronic condition risks, including T2D-related complications.

Preliminary investigations into the DiabeteBalance Diet have shown promising outcomes in T2D management, with improved blood sugar control, weight loss, and diminished dependence on diabetes medications.

Though additional long-term, randomized controlled trials are warranted to conclusively affirm the DiabeteBalance Diet's efficacy, the existing evidence offers an encouraging basis for appreciating this dietary strategy's potential advantages for those with T2D.

PART IV
MASTERING MEAL
PLANNING FOR BETTER
GLUCOSE CONTROL

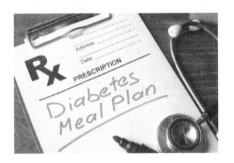

PERSONALIZING YOUR MEAL PLAN

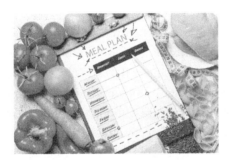

The DiabeteBalance Diet's comprehensive meal plan is a meticulously designed strategy that optimizes blood glucose control, enhances insulin sensitivity, aids weight loss, and decreases diabetes-related risks. By merging the 14 principles of the DiabeteBalance Diet with beneficial aspects of the Mediterranean and Glycemic Load diets, it addresses their limitations and provides a clear guide for food choices.

The integrated approach of the DiabeteBalance Diet encompasses healthy nutrition, lifestyle factors, and overall well-being, ensuring that all critical aspects of the Mediterranean Diet and Glycemic

Index-Glycemic Load diets for optimally managing diabetes are covered. By leveraging the health benefits of Mediterranean and Glycemic Load diets, such as improved heart health and glycemic control, the DiabeteBalance Diet maximizes its effectiveness.

The DiabeteBalance Diet focuses on incorporating low glycemic load, whole, and nutrient-rich foods such as raw fruits, raw vegetables, whole grains, lean proteins, and healthy fats like olive oil. It addresses common blind spots, including the impact of careless fruit consumption on blood sugar levels and the potential weight gain resulting from a lack of portion control.

KEY FEATURES OF THE COMPREHENSIVE MEAL PLANNING APPROACH:

- **Glycemic Index and Glycemic Load:** The DiabeteBalance Diet places a significant emphasis on understanding and utilizing the glycemic index (GI) and glycemic load (GL) of foods. This knowledge empowers individuals to achieve better blood sugar control, support weight loss, and reduce the risk of diabetes-related complications. Practical guidance is provided, including ranking foods based on their GI, GL, serving size, and net carbs, enabling informed food choices that foster improved insulin sensitivity, weight management, and overall health.
- **Mediterranean Diet Influence:** The meal planning approach draws inspiration from the renowned Mediterranean diet, which emphasizes heart-healthy fats, lean proteins, and a diverse array of fruits, vegetables, and whole grains. This dietary pattern has been linked with lower diabetes rates and improved glycemic control, making it an ideal foundation for the DiabeteBalance Diet.
- **Weight Management:** Weight loss, achieved through a caloric deficit, is a crucial aspect of reversing T2D. Effective weight

management leads to improved blood sugar control and significantly reduces the risk of diabetes-related complications. The DiabeteBalance Diet provides strategies and recommendations to support successful weight management.

- **Comorbidity Management:** The DiabeteBalance Diet addresses comorbid illnesses commonly associated with diabetes, such as hypertension and heart disease. It offers dietary recommendations that cater to these conditions, promoting a holistic approach to managing overall health and reducing the risk of complications.

- **Prevention of Life-threatening Complications:** By managing blood glucose levels through a nutrient-rich diet, the DiabeteBalance Diet significantly reduces the likelihood of severe complications such as kidney disease, nerve damage, heart disease, and stroke. It empowers individuals to take control of their health and mitigate the risks associated with diabetes.

- **Personalization and Flexibility:** The DiabeteBalance Diet encourages customization based on individual needs, food preferences, and lifestyle factors. It provides a flexible structure or framework that can be adapted to various situations and requirements, ensuring that individuals can tailor their meal plans to suit their unique circumstances.

- **Integration of Latest Nutritional Guidelines:** The meal planning approach aligns with the 2020-2025 Dietary Guidelines for Americans, emphasizing the consumption of a variety of nutrient-dense foods while limiting added sugars, saturated fats, and sodium intake. By incorporating these latest nutritional guidelines, the DiabeteBalance Diet ensures that individuals receive optimal nutrition for their health and well-being.

- **Addressing Psychological Aspects of Eating:** The DiabeteBalance Diet recognizes and addresses the psychological aspects of eating, including emotional eating triggers and the importance of mindful eating. It emphasizes the development of a healthier relationship with food, acknowledging that psychological factors can significantly influence dietary choices.

Overall, the DiabeteBalance Diet provides a powerful tool for managing diabetes, promoting weight loss, and improving overall health. It offers a sustainable and flexible dietary lifestyle that supports long-term well-being.

Creating Your Personalized Meal Plan

Creating a tailored meal plan is critical for effective diabetes management and weight loss. It should reflect your health goals, food preferences, and lifestyle while balancing essential nutrients to support diabetes optimal management efforts. Here's an extended and improved version of the plan:

- **Define Your Health Goals and Dietary Preferences:** Clearly set your goals, like weight loss or improved blood glucose control. Consider any dietary restrictions or personal food preferences you have, such as vegetarian or gluten-free. Also, take into account your daily routine and available meal preparation time. This will help you create a meal plan that fits seamlessly into your lifestyle.
- **Embrace the Principles of the Mediterranean Diet:** Ensure your meal plan includes a variety of vegetables, fruits, lean proteins, whole grains, and heart-healthy fats like olive oil. These elements are central to the Mediterranean diet, which is associated with improved health outcomes, including better glycemic control. The Mediterranean diet's emphasis on whole foods and plant-based ingredients provides a solid foundation for a diabetes-friendly meal plan.

- **Incorporate Low Glycemic Index (GI) and Glycemic Load (GL) Foods:** Diversify your diet with a range of low GI and GL foods. These foods have a smaller impact on blood sugar levels compared to high GI foods. Check the GI and GL values of foods when available to make informed choices. By including low GI and GL foods like non-starchy vegetables, legumes, whole grains, and berries, you can aid keep stable blood glucose levels and promote better overall glycemic control.

- **Prioritize Weight Loss:** Weight loss plays a significant role in managing diabetes. Achieve a caloric deficit by implementing portion control strategies and including low-calorie, nutrient-dense foods. Focus on incorporating more vegetables, lean proteins, and whole grains while minimizing high-calorie foods. This will help you create a meal plan that supports weight loss while providing essential nutrients for optimal health.

- **Integrate the 14 principles of the DiabeteBalance Diet:** The 14 principles of the DiabeteBalance Diet provide a comprehensive framework for food choices, meal timing, and nutrient balance. These principles encompass aspects such as portion control, food quality, and timing strategies to optimize blood glucose control and promote weight loss. By following these principles, you can ensure that your meal plan is well-rounded and effective in effectively managing diabetes.

- **Regulate Meal Frequency and Timing:** Consistent meal times and frequency are crucial for blood glucose control and weight management. Strive for consistent meal timings and consider incorporating smaller, more frequent meals throughout the day. This approach helps in maintaining stable blood glucose levels, preventing excessive food intake, and promoting overall satiety.

- **Balance Macronutrients:** Regulate your intake of carbohydrates, proteins, and fats to support blood glucose control and weight management. Include low-GI carbohydrates, lean proteins, and heart-healthy fats in your meals. Strive for a well-balanced plate that includes a variety of nutrients. By combining carbohydrates with proteins or fats, you can effectively slow down the absorption of sugars into the bloodstream.

- **Plan for Special Situations:** Be prepared for situations like dining out, managing other health conditions, or adjusting plans for physical activity. Research restaurant menus in advance to make healthier choices. Consult your healthcare team for guidance on managing comorbid conditions effectively, as they can provide tailored recommendations. Adjust your meals based on the intensity and duration of physical activities to maintain stable blood glucose levels and ensure proper fueling for exercise.

By aligning your meal plan with your unique needs and integrating Mediterranean diet principles and the 14 principles of the Diabete-Balance Diet, you can create a sustainable and effective path toward effectively managing diabetes.

CRAFTING YOUR ESSENTIAL SHOPPING LIST FOR THE TYPE 2 DIABETES OPTIMAL DIET

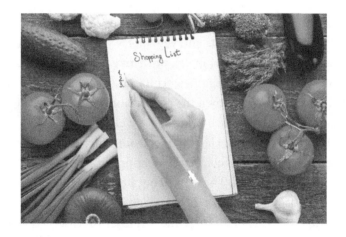

Starting a balanced, sustainable diet to optimally manage diabetes might feel like a challenge, especially when faced with many grocery store options. But, with a cleverly planned shopping list, you can make healthier choices more easily, stick to the DiabeteBalance Diet's rules, and meet your health and weight loss goals. Here are some simple tips to get you started:

- **Planning Ahead:** A good diet starts with good planning.

Make a shopping list before you go to the store to avoid buying things you don't need. Each week, set aside some time to plan meals and snacks that will aid you reach your diet and weight loss goals.

- **Choosing Whole Foods:** When making your shopping list, focus on fresh, whole foods that are part of the DiabeteBalance Diet. These include lean proteins, Low-GI whole grains, fruits, vegetables, and healthy fats, which help keep you healthy and your blood sugar levels stable.
- **Mixing Up Your Proteins:** Lean proteins are a key part of the DiabeteBalance Diet. Your shopping list should include both animal-based proteins like chicken, turkey, fish, eggs, and Greek yogurt, as well as plant-based proteins like legumes, tofu, and lentils. These proteins provide essential nutrients without too many unhealthy fats or calories.
- **Going for Low-GL and Fiber-Rich Foods:** Make sure to include a variety of fruits and vegetables with low Glycemic Load (GL) values. Additionally, prioritize fiber-rich foods such as whole grains, legumes, fruits, and vegetables. These foods aid in slowing down the absorption of carbohydrates, promoting more stable blood sugar levels.
- **Adding Healthy Fats:** Healthy fats from sources like olive oil, avocados, nuts, and seeds play an important role in the DiabeteBalance Diet. These fats contain essential fatty acids and help balance your meals' glycemic index.
- **Cutting Out Sugary Drinks and Highly Processed Foods:** Replace sugary drinks and processed foods with whole foods, water, unsweetened coffee, or tea. This can help prevent spikes in your blood sugar levels.
- **Choosing Low-GL Snacks:** Keep a selection of healthy, low-GL snacks on hand for between meals. Nuts, seeds, and raw veggies with hummus are good options.
- **Navigating the Supermarket:** Generally, you'll find the freshest produce, lean proteins, and dairy products around the edges of the store. You can also try local farmers' markets or

ethnic grocery stores for a wider variety of fresh produce and whole grain products.

- **Checking Labels:** When buying packaged foods, look at nutrition labels for added sugars, sodium, and trans fats. This will help you make healthier choices.
- **Meal Prepping:** Prepare meals in advance and store them in portions for the week. This saves time and helps you avoid unhealthy convenience foods.
- **Staying Hydrated:** Remember to include water on your shopping list. You can also add unsweetened herbal teas or infused water for variety. Avoid sugary drinks like soda, sweetened drinks and fruit juice.
- **Using Herbs and Spices:** Add flavor to your meals with herbs, spices, and flavor enhancers like garlic, ginger, and fresh herbs. These can make your meals taste better and also have potential health benefits.
- **Making Smart Snack Choices:** Choose nutrient-rich snacks that are part of the DiabeteBalance Diet. Good options include unsalted nuts, seeds, Greek yogurt, and low-fat cheese.
- **Shopping Mindfully:** Be aware of portion sizes and avoid unnecessary temptations. Choose smaller packages or portioned options to help control portions.
- **Getting Support and Education:** Consider getting advice from a dietitian or diabetes educator. They can help you tailor your shopping list to your specific needs and answer questions about managing your diabetes through diet.
- **Monitoring and Adjusting:** Track your progress and adjust your shopping list as needed. Pay attention to how different foods affect your body and blood sugar levels.
- **Being Careful with "Diet" Products:** "Diet" or "low-fat" products often contain hidden sugars and artificial ingredients. Always verify the ingredient list and nutritional information and choose whole foods when possible.
- **Revising Traditional Recipes:** Try changing traditional

recipes to fit the DiabeteBalance Diet. Use healthier substitutes for ingredients that are high in sugars or unhealthy fats.

- **Shopping Seasonally:** Choose fruits and vegetables that are in season. They're usually fresher, more flavorful, and cheaper.
- **Trying New Foods and Recipes:** Experiment with new foods and recipes that follow the DiabeteBalance Diet. This can make your diet more interesting and sustainable.
- **Buying in Bulk:** Buying non-perishable items like whole grains, legumes, and nuts in bulk can save money and ensure you always have key ingredients on hand.
- **Budgeting:** Having a grocery budget can aid you prevent impulse buys and focus on the essentials. Prioritize nutrient-dense foods that provide more health benefits.
- **Shopping Online:** If possible, consider online grocery shopping. It lets you take your time, carefully read product descriptions, and avoid in-store temptations.
- **Rotating Meals:** Avoid getting bored with your diet by rotating different meals that follow the DiabeteBalance Diet.
- **Making Smooth Transitions:** Make changes to your shopping list and meals gradually. This will make it easier to stick to your new diet.
- **Celebrating Progress:** Lastly, remember to celebrate your progress. Even small achievements can help motivate you to keep up your healthy eating habits.

With these simple strategies, you can navigate toward a balanced and sustainable diet for optimally managing diabetes.

COOKING TECHNIQUES AND PREPARATION

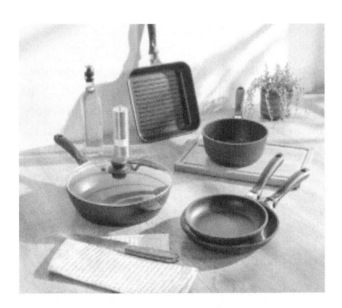

Embarking on a journey toward a balanced and sustainable diet for optimally managing Type 2 Diabetes requires careful consideration of both the foods we eat and how we prepare them. The twin cycle hypothesis highlights the importance of dietary choices and cooking methods in reducing fat stores in the pancreas and liver, a key aspect of optimally managing diabetes. By adhering to the principles of the DiabeteBalance Diet, optimizing cooking techniques, and focusing on reducing the Glycemic Index (GI) and Glycemic Load (GL) of meals, we can effectively manage and potentially reverse diabetes.

Let's delve into the pros and cons of various cooking techniques that align with the DiabeteBalance Diet principles and support your efforts in optimally managing diabetes:

Baking:

- Pros: Minimal added fat, making it ideal for preparing lean meats, fish, poultry, vegetables, and whole-grain dishes.
- Cons: Extended cooking times and high temperatures may lead to the loss of some water-soluble vitamins.

Broiling:

- Pros: Creates a flavorful crust while retaining moisture, suitable for lean proteins and vegetables.
- Cons: Cooking meat at high temperatures can produce potentially harmful substances like heterocyclic amines (HCAs) and polycyclic aromatic hydrocarbons (PAHs).

Grilling:

- Pros: Imparts a unique, smoky flavor and cooks food quickly with minimal added fat. Ideal for lean meats, fish, vegetables, and fruits.
- Cons: Similar to broiling, grilling meat at high temperatures can produce HCAs and PAHs.

Poaching:

- Pros: Requires no added fat and helps retain nutrients,

making it perfect for delicate proteins like fish, eggs, and poultry.

- Cons: Poaching may result in dishes that are less flavorful compared to other cooking methods. Consider using seasoned poaching liquids to enhance taste.

Roasting:

- Pros: Cooks food evenly and develops rich flavors, making it ideal for meats, poultry, and vegetables.
- Cons: Extended cooking times and high temperatures may lead to the loss of some nutrients.

Pressure Cooking:

- Pros: Reduces cooking times and helps retain nutrients. Ideal for legumes, whole grains, and tenderizing tough cuts of meat.
- Cons: Improper use can lead to overcooked or undercooked food, and pressure cooking can be intimidating for some users.

Slow Cooking:

- Pros: Requires minimal hands-on time and develops deep, complex flavors. Perfect for soups, stews, and tenderizing tough cuts of meat.
- Cons: Extended cooking times and high temperatures may result in the loss of some nutrients.

Stir-frying or Sautéing:

- Pros: Cooks food quickly over high heat, helping retain nutrients and develop vibrant flavors. Ideal for vegetables, lean proteins, and whole grains.

- Cons: Requires some oil or fat, which can increase the calorie content of a dish. Always use heart-healthy oils in moderation.

Steaming:

- Pros: Requires no added fat and helps retain nutrients and moisture. Ideal for vegetables, fish, and shellfish.
- Cons: Steamed dishes may lack the depth of flavor associated with other cooking methods.

No-Cook:

- Pros: Helps conserve the maximum amount of nutrients in food. No-cook recipes often include raw fruits, vegetables, and simple salads.
- Cons: No-cook recipes may not be as filling or satisfying as cooked dishes.

In addition to cooking techniques, proactive meal planning and preparation play significant roles in the DiabeteBalance Diet. By incorporating the following strategies, you can improve blood glucose control, facilitate weight loss, and make substantial strides toward optimally managing diabetes:

- Weekly meal planning: Design a meal plan for the week ahead, incorporating the principles of the Mediterranean diet and the DiabeteBalance Diet. This involves including an assortment of low-GI foods, lean sources of protein, healthy fats, and low-GL fruits and vegetables.
- Shopping list preparation: Develop a detailed shopping list based on your meal plan to stay organized and avoid impulse purchases of high-GI foods.
- Scheduled meal prep time: Dedicate specific times each week

for meal preparation. This strategy eases the cooking process, ensuring you always have healthy, diet-appropriate meals ready.

- Prepare ingredients in advance: To simplify meal prep, wash, chop, and store fruits and vegetables ahead of time. Consider pre-cooking whole grains like brown rice or quinoa for easy use throughout the week.

To further streamline your meal preparation and align with the DiabeteBalance Diet principles, you can explore the practice of batch cooking. By preparing large quantities of food in advance, you can save time, reduce the temptation for unhealthy convenience foods, and lower stress.

Investing in the right kitchen tools and appliances can also enhance your meal preparation experience. Consider acquiring tools that facilitate efficient cooking and promote healthier food choices.

By applying these cooking techniques, meal planning strategies, and utilizing appropriate kitchen tools, you will create delicious, nutrient-dense, and low-GI meals. This not only facilitates blood glucose control and weight loss but also promotes the potential reversal of T2D.

GUIDELINES FOR VEGETABLES AND VEGETABLE PRODUCTS

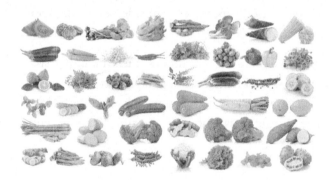

In the journey toward optimally managing diabetes, the role of vegetables cannot be overstated. These nutrient-dense powerhouses with their low glycemic index (GI) and high fiber content are at the core of the DiabeteBalance Diet. By incorporating these vegetables into your meals, you can enhance your health and maintain your blood glucose levels stable.

The DiabeteBalance Diet combines principles from the GI-GL approach, Mediterranean diet, and Dietary Guidelines for Americans 2020-2025. It categorizes foods into five distinct groups, with a significant emphasis on vegetables. These groups provide a roadmap for daily nutrition, ensuring you consume a well-rounded mix of macro and micronutrients.

Low-glycemic load vegetables, particularly non-starchy and low-carbohydrate ones like broccoli, asparagus, artichokes, and beets, are a substantial part of this diet. By focusing on foods with a low glycemic load, you can better manage and even reverse T2D.

These vegetables are rich in phytochemicals, vitamins, fiber, and minerals, making them incredibly beneficial for individuals with diabetes. For example, green leafy are packed with vitamin C and antioxidants, essential for managing diabetes.

Studies have shown that incorporating a diet high in low-glycemic load vegetables offers numerous health benefits. These include weight loss, improved insulin sensitivity, and lower Hemoglobin A1c (HbA1c) levels, a vital marker of long-term blood glucose control.

To confidently select, portion, and prepare these vegetables, it's essential to understand their significant role in your diet and how to integrate them effectively into your meals. This understanding will optimize their health benefits and bring you closer to your goal of optimally managing diabetes.

To start, correct portion sizes form the foundation of meal planning. **A single serving of vegetables typically comprises 1 cup of raw vegetables or salad, ½ cup of cooked vegetables, and ¾ to 1 cup (6-8 oz) of unsweetened, homemade vegetable juice.** Adjust these servings according to your appetite, caloric needs, and weight loss aspirations.

Strive for up to 10 daily servings across the five vegetable subgroups. This includes 1-2 servings of "Dark-Green Vegetables," 1-2 servings of "Red & Orange Vegetables," 1-2 servings of "Beans, Peas, Lentils," 2-3 servings of "Starchy Vegetables," and 2-3 servings of "Other Vegetables." A diverse intake ensures a comprehensive nutrient profile, leading to superior weight loss and blood glucose control outcomes.

Understanding the impact of cooking on the glycemic index (GI) of vegetables is crucial. Different cooking methods can alter the GI by changing the structure and availability of carbohydrates. Here's how various cooking methods affect the GI:

- Boiling and Steaming: These methods maintain the low-GI value of vegetables by softening the fiber without significantly altering carbohydrate structure. Avoid overcooking, as it can raise the GI.
- Roasting and Grilling: These methods may slightly increase the GI due to caramelization, but the effect is typically negligible. Roasted and grilled vegetables can still be an excellent component of a healthy, low-GI diet when used judiciously.
- Baking: Baking can slightly elevate the GI of starchy vegetables like potatoes. However, this increase doesn't categorize these foods as high-GI.
- Microwaving: Microwaving can marginally raise the GI of some vegetables, but the effect is minimal as it leads to minimal caramelization.
- Frying: Frying can considerably increase the GI of vegetables by altering the food structure, allowing faster carbohydrate absorption. Frying often incorporates fats or oils, increasing the overall calorie content.

Interestingly, the cooling of certain foods after boiling, like potatoes, pasta, and rice, triggers a process called retrogradation, which slows down digestion and lowers the GI.

To increase your vegetable intake and improve blood sugar control, consider the following strategies:

- Adding More Vegetables to Mixed Dishes: Incorporate extra vegetables into dishes you already enjoy, such as pasta, by adding bell peppers, onions, zucchini, or spinach to the sauce.

- Incorporating Vegetables into Breakfast: Change your breakfast routine by adding spinach or other greens to scrambled eggs or creating a vegetable hash with sweet potatoes, bell peppers, and onions.
- Blending Vegetables into Smoothies: Increase your vegetable intake by adding leafy greens like kale and spinach or vegetables like zucchini and cauliflower to your smoothies without significantly altering the taste.
- Preparing Vegetable-Based Sauces and Soups: Enjoy the benefits of a variety of vegetables in one meal by making vegetable soups or using marinara sauce with bell peppers, onions, and carrots.
- Opting for Fresh or Frozen Vegetables: Fresh and frozen vegetables are optimal choices for a healthy diet as they are typically free of added sugars and sodium. Frozen vegetables are a fantastic alternative when fresh ones aren't available or affordable.
- Pairing Vegetables with Protein and Healthy Fats: Including a protein source and healthy fats with your meals helps regulate blood sugar levels and makes your meals more satisfying, promoting weight loss by preventing overeating.
- Using the Food List: Utilize a detailed food list that provides the GI, GL, and carb values for various foods. This can help you make informed decisions about which vegetables to include in your meals and how best to prepare them.
- Vegetable Product Innovation: Explore vegetable-based products like spiralized vegetable noodles or cauliflower rice to add variety to your meals while maintaining blood sugar control and supporting weight loss efforts.

Remember, consistency is key. Start by making small changes to your diet, and over time, these changes will become healthier habits. By embracing the power of vegetables and incorporating them into your daily meals, you can take significant steps toward optimally managing diabetes.

GUIDELINES FOR FRUITS AND FRUIT PRODUCTS

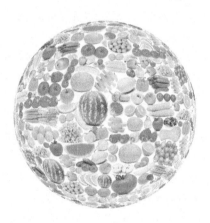

Fruits, much like vegetables, are crucial to The DiabeteBalance Diet. They're generally rich in fiber and essential nutrients and typically have low to moderate GI values. Incorporating them into your meal plans can significantly contribute to optimal blood glucose control, overall health, and sustainable weight loss.

UNDERSTANDING FRUIT PORTIONS:

It's vital to understand the correct portion sizes for fruits. A serving of fruit typically equates to one medium piece, 1 cup of sliced fruits, or ½ cup (4 oz) of fruit juice.

Here are some general guidelines for what counts as a serving of fruit:

- Fresh fruit: A serving size is generally about the size of a tennis ball or your fist. That's equivalent to a small apple, orange, or peach, or about 1/2 of a large banana.
- Berries or cherries: A serving is 1 cup.
- Grapes: A serving is about 15 grapes.
- Dried fruit: Because drying fruit removes water and concentrates sugars, a serving size is smaller. For example, 2 tablespoons of raisins or dried cranberries is a serving.
- Fruit Juice: Be careful with fruit juice, as it can have a lot of sugar and it doesn't contain the beneficial fiber found in whole fruit. A serving is 1/2 cup.
- Canned or frozen fruit: For canned fruit, a serving size is 1/2 cup. Choose canned fruit that's packed in water or its own juice, not syrup. For frozen fruit, a serving is also typically 1/2 cup.

DAILY FRUIT INTAKE:

Strive to consume 2 to 4 servings of fruits daily. To maximize fiber intake and promote weight loss, at least 60% of your total fruit intake should come from whole fruits rather than 100% juice. When choosing juices, opt for those without added sugars or food additives.

UNDERSTANDING FRUIT RIPENESS:

The ripeness of a fruit can significantly influence its GL. As fruits ripen, their sugar content increases, thus raising their GI and GL.

Therefore, less ripe fruits tend to have a lower GI. For instance, an unripe banana has a lower GI than a ripe one.

STRATEGIES TO INCREASE FRUIT INTAKE:

Here are some strategies to increase your fruit intake while improving blood sugar control:

- **Regular Consumption of Fruits:** Aim to include at least one serving of fruit in each of your meals. This doesn't necessarily mean eating a whole piece of fruit - it could be a handful of berries in your yogurt, slices of apple on your salad, or a side of melon with your dinner.
- **Adding Fruits to Breakfast:** Incorporating fruits into breakfast can make the meal more enjoyable while boosting its nutritional value. Add berries to your oatmeal, slices of banana to your cereal, or chopped fruit to your pancake batter. Avocado is a great addition to toast or eggs if you prefer savory breakfasts.
- **Choosing Whole Fruits as Snacks:** Whole fruits make excellent snacks as they're nutrient-rich, satisfying, and convenient. They provide fiber, which slows down the digestion of sugars and aids in keeping blood sugar levels stable. It's generally better to eat fruit whole rather than juiced to take full advantage of its fiber content.
- **Blending Fruits into Smoothies:** Similar to vegetables, you can effortlessly incorporate fruits into your diet by incorporating them into smoothies. This can be a fun and tasty way to consume a variety of fruits. To balance the sugar content, include a source of protein (e.g., Greek yogurt, protein powder) and healthy fats, like chia seeds or nut butter, in your smoothie.
- **Carrying Fruit for Later Consumption:** One of the biggest challenges when trying to eat more fruits is convenience. You can have a healthy snack readily available when hunger strikes

by simply carrying a piece of fruit with you, such as an apple or banana.

- Finding the Perfect Pairings with Your Favorite Foods: Fruits can also be paired with other foods to create satisfying meals or snacks. Pair apple slices with low-sodium cheese, spread nut butter on banana slices, or mix chopped fruit into cottage cheese or yogurt. Pairing fruit with a protein and/or fat source slows digestion and absorption of fruit sugars, which can aid maintain your blood sugar levels stable.

It's important to note that while fruits are nutritious, they do contain natural sugars and should be consumed as part of a balanced diet. Paying attention to portion sizes, especially for fruits that are higher in sugar or glycemic index, can help manage blood sugar levels effectively. By following these strategies and being mindful of your dietary needs and preferences, you can incorporate fruits into your The DiabeteBalance Diet in a way that supports blood sugar control and overall health.

CHOOSING THE RIGHT FRUITS:

Prioritize fruits with a lower GI. Berries, cherries, peaches, apricots, apples, oranges, and pears are excellent choices for weight loss. Limit high-GI fruits like ripe bananas, pineapples, and watermelons.

CHOOSE WHOLE FRUITS OVER JUICES:

Whole fruits have more fiber and a lower GI than fruit juices. This makes them better for blood sugar control and weight management. If you choose to have juice, ensure it's 100% fruit juice, and limit your serving size to 4 ounces.

FRESH OR FROZEN FRUITS ARE BEST:

Fresh and frozen fruits with no added sugars are your optimal choice. If using canned or dried fruits, look for options with no added sugar, and adjust portion sizes, as these forms are more concentrated and could lead to excessive caloric intake.

PAIR FRUITS WITH PROTEIN OR HEALTHY FATS:

To slow glucose absorption and avoid blood sugar spikes, pair your fruits with a source of protein or healthy fats. This can also enhance satiety, supporting weight loss. For example, pair apple slices with a handful of nuts or serve berries with a portion of Greek yogurt.

USE THE EXTENSIVE FOOD LIST:

The food list provided in this book, which includes GI, GL, Net Carb values, is an invaluable tool for making informed decisions about which fruits and fruit products to include in your diet and in what quantities.

EXPERIMENT WITH FRUIT PRODUCTS:

Low-sugar fruit products, such as unsweetened applesauce or fruit spreads, can add variety to your diet, making it more enjoyable and sustainable. Always check the labels for added sugars to ensure they align with your weight loss goals.

GUIDELINES FOR GRAINS

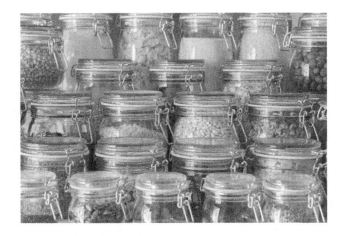

Grains are an important food group to consider when aiming to reverse diabetes, and their selection and consumption require careful thought. By taking into account factors such as the Glycemic Index (GI), Glycemic Load (GL), the principles of MedDiet, and the Dietary Guidelines for Americans 2020-2025, you can make informed choices about incorporating grains into your diet.

The Mediterranean diet places value on grains, particularly whole grains, due to their high dietary fiber, vitamin, mineral, and phytonu-trient content. They contribute to balanced nutrition and overall health promotion. However, not all grains provide equal benefits when it comes to diabetes optimal management.

Refined grains, which have undergone a milling process that removes their bran and germ, lose a significant amount of their nutritional value. White rice, white bread, and many processed cereals fall into this category. These products have high GI and GL values, leading to rapid blood glucose spikes, which can pose challenges for diabetes effective management.

Even certain whole grains like brown rice or whole wheat bread, while nutritionally superior to refined grains, may still have medium to high GI values. If not portioned appropriately or balanced with other foods, they can still cause blood sugar surges.

Integrating the principles of the Mediterranean diet with the GI-GL framework is crucial for effective diabetes management. The Diabete-Balance Diet combines these principles cohesively, addressing poten-tial pitfalls and providing a comprehensive strategy for optimally managing diabetes.

Understanding the carbohydrate content and portion sizes of grains is vital for diabetes meal planning. In the DiabeteBalance Diet, a serving of grains is typically equivalent to 15 grams of carbohydrates, and precise portion control is emphasized.

Given a target Glycemic Load (GL) of 50, which corresponds to 50 grams of pure glucose, it's important to carefully measure and control the amount of grains consumed.

This chapter aims to empower individuals to navigate the world of grains strategically. By understanding the differences among grain types, their GI and GL values, and how they fit into a balanced diet aimed at optimally managing diabetes, individuals can enjoy the bene-fits of grains while effectively managing potential concerns and confi-dently progressing on the path to optimally managing diabetes.

When choosing breakfast cereals, opt for options made from whole grains that are low in sugar and high in fiber. Many breakfast cereals can be high in added sugars, which can increase their GI and hinder weight loss efforts. Reading nutrition labels will assist in making informed choices.

To balance the impact of grains on blood sugar levels, pair them with a source of protein and healthy fats. This combination can slow down glucose absorption, prevent blood sugar spikes, promote satiety, and support weight loss. For example, consider having a slice of whole-grain bread with avocado and eggs for a nutritious and balanced breakfast.

The extensive food list provided in the book offers essential information such as the GI, GL values, serving sizes, and net carb content. Utilizing this resource empowers individuals to make informed decisions when including grains and breakfast cereals in their diet, helping them determine appropriate quantities for optimal weight management and overall well-being.

Understanding Portion Sizes:

Understanding and carefully measuring portion sizes is crucial in the DiabeteBalance Diet. The following serving sizes are recommended for cereals and grains:

Typical serving sizes for cereals and grains include:

- ⅓ cup of breakfast cereal or muesli.
- ½ cup of cooked cereal or other cooked grain.
- ⅓ cup of cooked rice (excluding white rice).
- ½ cup of cold cereal.

It's important to note that all breakfast cereals on the provided list are low-glycemic-index and support a healthy weight.

Balancing and variety are important for your daily grain intake. Aim for up to 3 servings per day, depending on your individual needs.

Strategies to increase your intake of whole grains could involve replacing white bread with whole grain bread, incorporating whole grains into salads or as a side dish, and choosing breakfast cereals made from whole grains. The goal is to incorporate grains to support blood glucose control, overall health, and weight loss.

By selecting the right grains, controlling portion sizes, and utilizing the provided food list, you can benefit from grains and breakfast cereals in a GI-focused diet while maintaining blood sugar control, supporting overall health, and promoting sustainable weight loss.

GUIDELINES FOR DAIRY AND PLANT-BASED ALTERNATIVES

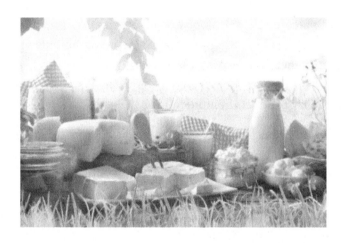

When meal planning for the DiabeteBalance Diet, it's crucial to understand the serving sizes of dairy products and their plant-based counterparts. This diverse food category includes traditional dairy items like milk, cheese, and yogurt, as well as plant-based alternatives such as soy, almond, and other non-dairy options. Incorporating dairy and its plant-based alternatives into your diet is essential for managing weight, controlling blood sugar, and improving overall health. These food choices align with important principles like the

Glycemic Index (GI), Glycemic Load (GL), the Mediterranean diet (MedDiet), and the Dietary Guidelines for Americans 2020-2025.

Scientific research has highlighted the potential advantages of dairy products, especially low-fat dairy, and yogurt, in optimally managing diabetes. Esteemed journals have published studies suggesting a correlation between higher intake of low-fat dairy and improved insulin sensitivity, reduced T2D risk, and better cardiometabolic profiles. However, it's essential to distinguish between various dairy products, as not all are beneficial in preventing T2D. Specifically, it seems that low-fat dairy foods, particularly yogurt, provide the most benefits, while other dairy items exhibit no clear association.

Milk and other dairy items usually have a low glycemic load (GL) due to the moderate GI effect of lactose and the capacity of milk protein to slow down stomach emptying. This combination leads to a gradual release of glucose into the bloodstream, causing less impact on blood sugar levels compared to high-GI foods. Including suitable servings of dairy in the diet can lead to improved glycemic control, aiding in diabetes management. Remember to be aware of portion sizes and consume dairy products in moderation.

Dairy consumption also plays a significant role in weight management, a critical component of the DiabeteBalance Diet. When consumed in moderation and paired with regular exercise, low-fat dairy products can support weight loss goals. Furthermore, dairy products align with the principles of MedDiet, which promotes the consumption of low-fat dairy products. These products provide essential nutrients like calcium and protein, contributing to overall health and well-being.

However, what about plant-based alternatives? In addition to dairy products, plant-based alternatives play a crucial role in the Diabete-Balance Diet. These alternatives offer choices for individuals who prefer to limit or avoid dairy, have lactose intolerance, or follow a plant-based lifestyle. Plant-based alternatives include soy milk, almond milk, coconut milk, oat milk, and other non-dairy options.

In the context of optimally managing diabetes, plant-based alternatives have several benefits. They typically contain lower amounts of saturated fat and cholesterol compared to traditional dairy products, which can be advantageous for cardiovascular health. Fortified plant-based milk alternatives can provide similar essential nutrients as dairy milk. Moreover, plant-based alternatives align with the principles of MedDiet and the Dietary Guidelines for Americans, which emphasize the inclusion of diverse protein sources, including plant-based options. Incorporating plant-based milk alternatives, along with other plant-based proteins like legumes, nuts, and seeds, supports a well-rounded diet that promotes overall health and aids in diabetes management.

When selecting plant-based alternatives for The DiabeteBalance Diet, it is important to focus on minimally processed options without added sugars. Reading labels and opting for unsweetened or low-sugar varieties is recommended. Additionally, ensuring adequate intake of nutrients typically found in dairy products, like calcium and vitamin D, can be achieved by choosing fortified plant-based alternatives or incorporating other dietary sources of these nutrients.

A critical point to remember, whether you choose dairy products or plant-based alternatives, is the importance of understanding serving sizes. The sugar content of these foods can vary significantly. Traditional dairy products naturally contain a type of sugar known as lactose, while plant-based alternatives often contain added sugars (e.g., cane sugar, rice syrup) or other sweeteners to enhance their flavor. Therefore, a serving size must correspond to 15 grams of carbohydrates, aligning with the principles of carbohydrate counting in diabetes management.

Understanding Serving Sizes:

Becoming familiar with the typical serving sizes for dairy products and plant-based alternatives can help manage your carbohydrate intake and control blood glucose levels. Remember, for the purposes of carbohydrate counting in diabetes management, a serving size should correspond to a food containing 15 grams of carbohydrates.

Dairy Products:

- Milk: A typical serving size is one cup (8 ounces). This serving size of milk, whether whole, low-fat, or non-fat, contains approximately 12 grams of carbohydrates, all from lactose, the natural sugar in milk.
- Cheese: For hard cheeses, a typical serving size is 1.5 ounces, and these usually contain minimal to no carbohydrates. For soft cheeses like cottage cheese, a serving size is typically half a cup, containing about 4-6 grams of carbohydrates.
- Yogurt: For plain yogurt, a serving size is typically one cup, with approximately 10 grams of carbohydrates in non-fat yogurt and 16 grams in low-fat yogurt. Be cautious with flavored or sweetened yogurts, as these can contain significantly more carbohydrates.

Plant-Based Alternatives:

- Almond Milk: A typical serving size is one cup, which generally contains just 1-2 grams of carbohydrates for the unsweetened variety.
- Soy Milk: A typical one-cup serving of unsweetened soy milk contains about 4 grams of carbohydrates.
- Other Alternatives: For other plant-based milks like oat, rice, or coconut milk, a serving size is one cup. However, the carbohydrate content can vary widely.
- Unsweetened oat milk contains about 16 grams of carbohydrates per serving, while rice milk can contain upwards of 20-25 grams. Unsweetened coconut milk typically contains fewer than 2 grams per serving.
- Tofu: For tofu, a typical serving size is 3 ounces, containing about 3 grams of carbohydrates.

While it is vital to consider the carbohydrate content, do not overlook the nutrient density of these food choices. Dairy products provide abundant protein, calcium, and vitamin D. Alternatively, plant-based alternatives can offer valuable fiber, especially those derived from legumes or nuts. When selecting products, it is essential to check food labels for the most accurate and up-to-date nutrient information.

It's also essential to consider the sodium content, especially in cheese and processed dairy products. High sodium intake contribute significantly to increased blood pressure, posing additional health concerns, particularly for individuals with diabetes who are already at an increased risk of cardiovascular disease. Always check the nutrition labels for sodium content and choose lower-sodium options whenever possible.

In terms of processing, remember that the least processed options are often the healthiest. Highly processed foods can contain a plethora of additives, artificial ingredients, and preservatives that may not align with the DiabeteBalance Diet. Opt for whole foods whenever possible and scrutinize labels to select minimally processed dairy products and plant-based alternatives.

Consider the following suggestions for incorporating dairy and non-dairy alternatives into The DiabeteBalance Diet:

- **Opt for Low-Fat and Non-Dairy Alternatives:** Choose low-fat or non-fat dairy products and fortified soy alternatives. These options generally have a lower glycemic index (GI) and can participate in weight loss and overall health. Opt for unsweetened versions whenever possible to avoid added sugars, which can interfere with both blood sugar control and weight management.
- **Consider Portion Sizes:** Controlling portion sizes is crucial for managing blood glucose levels and controlling calorie

intake to support weight loss. A typical serving size for dairy and fortified soy alternatives is 1 cup of milk, yogurt, or 1.5 ounces of cheese.

- **Pair Dairy with Other Foods:** Pairing dairy products with other foods can help slow the absorption of glucose, maintain steady blood sugar levels, and enhance satiety, which is beneficial for weight loss. For example, you could pair a cup of reduced-fat yogurt with a handful of nuts and seeds for a balanced snack.

- **Use the Food List:** Make use of the comprehensive food list provided in this guide. It includes information on glycemic index (GI), glycemic load (GL), and net carb values, helping you make informed decisions about which dairy products and fortified soy alternatives to include in your diet and in what quantities while supporting weight loss.

- **Daily Dairy Intake:** Aim for 2-3 servings of dairy or fortified alternatives per day. This quantity can be adjusted based on individual dietary needs, preferences, and weight loss goals.

- **Experiment with Dairy and Plant-based Alternatives:** Many different types of dairy products and fortified alternatives are available. Experimenting with these can add variety to your diet and make your meals more enjoyable while still contributing to weight loss.

- **Choose Fermented Dairy Products:** Incorporate fermented dairy products like yogurt and kefir into your diet. These products contain beneficial probiotics that support gut health and may have a positive impact on blood sugar control.

- **Explore Nut and Seed Milks:** In addition to soy milk, it's worth exploring the range of nut and seed milks available, such as almond milk, coconut milk, or hemp milk. These alternatives provide a variety of flavors and can be an adequate option for individuals with lactose intolerance or those following a plant-based lifestyle.

- **Incorporate Dairy and Alternatives into Recipes:** Look for recipes that incorporate dairy products or their alternatives.

For example, you can use Greek yogurt as a base for salad dressings or smoothies, or try using almond milk in your morning oatmeal. Experimenting with different recipes can help you discover new and enjoyable ways to include dairy and non-dairy alternatives in your meals.

- **Take into consideration Calcium and Vitamin D Supplements:** If you decide to restrict or eliminate dairy products and their alternatives from your diet, it's crucial to ensure you have an adequate intake of vitamin D and calcium, which are needed for maintaining strong and healthy bones. Consulting with your healthcare provider is recommended to determine if supplements are necessary to meet your specific nutritional requirements.

By incorporating dairy and non-dairy alternatives mindfully and in appropriate portion sizes, you can support your efforts in optimally managing diabetes.

GUIDELINES FOR PROTEIN FOODS

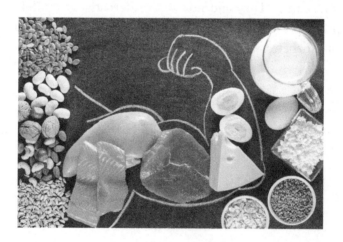

Transitioning to proteins is a crucial aspect of the DiabeteBalance Diet as they are essential nutrients that support various biological functions in the body. Both animal-based and plant-based proteins play important roles in maintaining steady blood glucose levels, aiding in weight loss, and promoting overall health. These principles align with the Glycemic Index (GI) - Glycemic Load (GL) framework, the Mediterranean Diet (MedDiet), and the Dietary Guidelines for Americans 2020-2025.

THE COMPLETE DIABETES FOOD ENCYCLOPEDIA

Understanding the different subcategories within the protein food group, their unique benefits, and potential risks is important. Animal proteins, such as chicken, beef, pork, fish, eggs, and dairy, are primary sources of protein. Plant proteins include legumes, nuts, seeds, and whole grains. Both animal and plant proteins have a place in the DiabeteBalance Diet, but finding the right balance is key.

Numerous studies have shown that incorporating a variety of plant proteins alongside lean animal proteins can lead to greater reductions in serum cholesterol. This underscores the significance of incorporating a diverse array of proteins, with a preference for plant-based sources, aligning with the principles of the MedDiet.

It's essential to approach a high-protein diet with caution. While it may potentially benefit by improving HbA1c and liver fat content, high protein intake can strain the kidneys, especially in individuals with pre-existing Chronic Kidney Disease (CKD), even in its early stages. Therefore, moderation and balance are essential when incorporating proteins into a diet aimed at optimally managing diabetes.

Recognizing the potential risks linked to inadequate protein intake is equally essential. Not consuming enough protein can result in adverse effects such as muscle loss, compromised immune function, and various health complications. These consequences can negatively impact diabetes management and overall health.

The goal is to provide comprehensive guidance on how to optimally include proteins in the diet. This involves understanding the correct balance of animal and plant proteins, appropriate portion sizes, the importance of choosing lean and low-fat options, and incorporating proteins in a way that manages blood glucose levels, supports weight loss, and enhances overall health. With this knowledge, you can make smart, informed choices to support the journey toward optimally managing diabetes.

Opt for Lean Proteins:

Select lean protein sources like chicken breast, turkey, fish, eggs, and plant-based proteins like lentils, chickpeas, and tofu. Typically, these choices offer a low glycemic index (GI) and are crucial for promoting weight loss and maintaining good health. Be mindful of cooking methods; opt for grilling, broiling, or steaming rather than frying to avoid unnecessary fats and calories.

Consider Portion Sizes:

A typical serving size for protein-rich foods is approximately 3 ounces (85 grams) of cooked meat, poultry, or fish, 1 egg, 1/2 cup (125 grams) of cooked beans, or 2 tablespoons of peanut butter. Controlling portion sizes is essential for managing blood glucose levels and controlling calorie intake to support weight loss.

Pair Protein with Other Foods:

Pairing protein-rich foods with other nutritious foods can help maintain steady blood sugar levels and enhance satiety, which is beneficial for weight loss. For example, you could pair a grilled chicken breast with a serving of quinoa and colorful vegetables for a balanced meal.

Use the Food List:

The comprehensive foods lists provided in this book not only include GI, GL, and net carb values but also account for various cooking and preparation methods that can impact the understanding of their effects. This detailed information allows you to make informed decisions about the protein-rich foods you include in your diet and consider how different cooking and preparation methods may influence their impact on blood sugar levels and weight loss efforts.

Daily Protein Intake:

Aim for 2-3 servings of protein-rich foods per day. This quantity can be adjusted based on individual dietary needs, preferences, and weight loss goals.

Experiment with Protein Sources:

Many different types of protein-rich foods are available, both animal-based and plant-based. Experimenting with these can add variety to your diet and make your meals more enjoyable while still contributing to weight loss.

These guidelines can help you enjoy the benefits of protein-rich foods while maintaining blood sugar control, supporting overall health, and promoting weight loss.

PART V
THE BEST FOODS

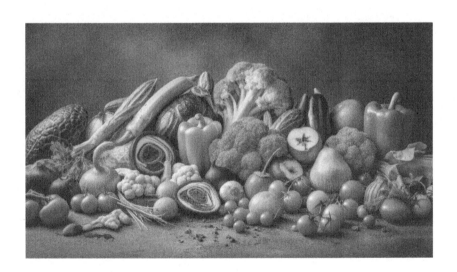

BREADS AND BAKED PRODUCTS

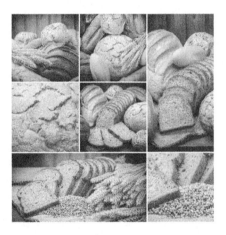

Bread and baked products are integral to many diets, including those targeted at optimally managing diabetes. Their role in such a diet must be considered carefully, with an emphasis on understanding their impact on glycemic load (GL) and how well they align with the objectives of the DiabeteBalance Diet. Knowledge of these foods' benefits and potential drawbacks allows for more informed dietary choices that bolster diabetes management and overall health.

Benefits of Breads and Baked Products:

- **Fiber-Rich**: Whole-grain bread and baked goods, including whole wheat bread, oatmeal cookies, and bran muffins, are rich sources of dietary fiber, facilitating a steady release of glucose into the bloodstream. This process helps mitigate sudden blood sugar spikes, improving glycemic control.
- **Nutrient-Dense**: Whole-grain bread and baked goods supply essential nutrients such as B-vitamins, iron, and magnesium. Compared to their refined white counterparts, these whole-grain options retain the nutrient-rich bran and germ of the grain. This nutrient density can help prevent deficiencies commonly associated with T2D and enhance overall health.
- **Promote Satiety and Portion Control**: Whole grains and seeds in bread and baked products can enhance satiety, helping curb appetite. Incorporating these foods in moderate amounts can assist with portion control, preventing overeating, and promoting weight management, a key aspect of diabetes management.

Drawbacks of Breads and Baked Products:

- **High Glycemic Load**: Refined grain bread and baked goods exhibit a high glycemic load, leading to an abrupt spike in blood sugar levels. This can be problematic for individuals with T2D. Therefore, opting for products with a lower glycemic load, like whole grain options or those made with alternative low-glycemic load flours such as almond or coconut, is advisable.
- **Added Sugars and Unhealthy Fats**: Commercially produced baked goods often contain high levels of added sugars and unhealthy fats. These elements can contribute to weight gain, increased insulin resistance, and higher blood sugar levels. It's crucial to scrutinize labels and choose products low in added sugars and trans fats.

- **Portion Control Challenges**: Even whole-grain bread and baked goods can be calorie-dense, making overconsumption easy and potentially leading to excess calorie intake. Practicing portion control and awareness of serving sizes can help mitigate this risk.

Incorporating Breads and Baked Products into The DiabeteBalance Diet:

To successfully include bread and baked products in your eating plan, consider the following:

- **Choose Whole Grains**: Prioritize whole grain bread, whole wheat tortillas, and other baked goods made with whole grain flour. Identify keywords like "whole wheat," "whole grain," or "100% whole" on product labels.
- **Monitor Glycemic Load**: Choose bread and baked goods with a lower glycemic load to minimize blood sugar spikes. Generally, whole grains have a lower glycemic load than refined grains.
- **Control Portion Sizes**: Avoid excessive calorie intake by keeping portions in check. Adhere to recommended serving sizes and consider using smaller plates or bowls to help maintain portion control.
- **Consider Homemade Options**: Baking at home provides the advantage of ingredient control, allowing you to reduce added sugars and unhealthy fats. Experiment with alternative flours such as almond, coconut, or whole wheat pastry flour to enhance the nutrient density and fiber content.
- **Adopt a Mediterranean Approach**: Incorporate bread and baked products with other elements of the Mediterranean diet, including vegetables, legumes, lean proteins, and healthy fats. This diet emphasizes whole foods and can help balance the glycemic load of a meal.

The following list provides a comprehensive selection of foods that fully comply with the DiabeteBalance Diet. Each entry includes crucial details such as serving size, Glycemic Index (GI), Glycemic Load (GL), and Net Carbohydrates. This information equips you with the knowledge needed to make informed decisions regarding portion sizes and effective meal planning. The foods are sorted alphabetically for easy reference.

LOW GLYCEMIC LOAD FOODS A-Z

▦ Almond Flour Bread , (1 slice, 25g): GI of 35, GL of 10.5, Net carb= 3g

▦ Barley Bread , (1 slice, 25g): GI of 34, GL of 4.1, Net carb= 12g

▦ Biscotti, (1 biscotti, 20g): GI of 40, GL of 8, Net carb= 12g

▦ Brioche, (1 slice, 30g): GI of 54, GL of 8, Net carb= 15g

▦ Buckwheat Bread , (1 slice, 25g): GI of 47, GL of 7, Net carb= 15g

▦ Butter Cookies, (1 cookie, 30g): GI of 50, GL of 7, Net carb= 11g

▦ Cheese and Herb Biscuits, (1 biscuit, 35g): GI of 62, GL of 5, Net carb= 13g

▦ Coconut Flour Bread, (1 slice, 25g): GI of 45, GL of 1, Net carb= 2g

▦ Coconut Macaroons, (1 macaroon, 20g): GI of 50, GL of 5, Net carb= 10g

▦ Corn Tortilla , (1 medium tortilla, 55g): GI of 52, GL of 6.8, Net carb= 13g

▦ Drop Biscuits, (1 biscuit, 30g): GI of 62, GL of 5, Net carb= 11g

▤ Ezekiel Bread, (1 slice, 25g): GI of 36, GL of 4.3, Net carb= 12g

▤ Flaxseed Bread, (1 slice, 25g): GI of 45, GL of 4.5, Net carb= 10g

▤ Garlic Butter Biscuits, (1 biscuit, 25g): GI of 62, GL of 3, Net carb= 10g

▤ Gluten-Free Multiseed Bread, (1 slice, 25g): GI of 50, GL of 5.5, Net carb= 11g

▤ Green Onion Biscuits, (1 biscuit, 28g): GI of 55, GL of 7, Net carb= 14g

▤ Italian Bread, (1 slice, 30g): GI of 70, GL of 10, Net carb= 14g

▤ Keto Bread , (1 slice, 25g): GI of 10, GL of 2, Net carb= 2g

▤ Lemon Cookies, (1 cookie, 30g): GI of 55, GL of 9, Net carb= 14g

▤ Low-Carb Tortilla , (1 medium tortilla, 55g): GI of 30, GL of 1.8, Net carb= 6g

▤ Oat Bread , (1 slice, 25g): GI of 55, GL of 8.3, Net carb= 15g

▤ Pão de Queijo, (1 piece, 30g): GI of 35, GL of 5, Net carb= 15g

▤ Peanut Butter Blossoms, (1 cookie, 30g): GI of 50, GL of 7, Net carb= 13g

▤ Peanut Butter Cookies, (1 cookie, 30g): GI of 50, GL of 7, Net carb= 13g

▤ Pesto Biscuits, (1 biscuit, 28g): GI of 65, GL of 8, Net carb= 15g

▤ Pumpernickel Bread, (1 slice, 30g): GI of 50, GL of 6, Net carb= 13g

▤ Pumpernickel Bread , (1 slice, 25g): GI of 50, GL of 6.5, Net carb= 13g

▤ Pumpkin Biscuits, (1 biscuit, 28g): GI of 70, GL of 9, Net carb= 15g

▤ Quiche, (1 slice, 100g): GI of 30, GL of 3, Net carb= 10g

▤ Quinoa Bread , (1 slice, 25g): GI of 53, GL of 7, Net carb= 13g

Raspberry Tart, (1 slice, 100g): GI of 65, GL of 6, Net carb= 15g

Rosemary Biscuits, (1 biscuit, 38g): GI of 62, GL of 6, Net carb= 15g

Rye Bread, (1 slice, 25g): GI of 50, GL of 7, Net carb= 14g

Rye Bread , (1 slice, 25g): GI of 58, GL of 8.1, Net carb= 14g

Shortbread Cookies, (1 cookie, 30g): GI of 50, GL of 7, Net carb= 11g

Snickerdoodle Cookies, (1 cookie, 30g): GI of 55, GL of 9, Net carb= 14g

Sourdough Bread, (1 slice, 30g): GI of 52, GL of 8, Net carb= 15g

Sourdough Bread , (1 slice, 25g): GI of 53, GL of 8, Net carb= 15g

Soy and Linseed Bread, (1 slice, 25g): GI of 27, GL of 2.7, Net carb= 10g

Spelt Bread , (1 slice, 25g): GI of 54, GL of 8.7, Net carb= 16g

Strudel, (1 slice, 100g): GI of 65, GL of 6, Net carb= 15g

Tres Leches Cake, (1 slice, 100g): GI of 25, GL of 6, Net carb= 10g

Wheat Tortilla, (1 medium tortilla, 55g): GI of 30, GL of 5.4, Net carb= 18g

Whole Grain Bread , (1 slice, 25g): GI of 51, GL of 6.1, Net carb= 12g

Whole Grain Ciabatta, (1 small roll, 25g): GI of 58, GL of 8.7, Net carb= 15g

Whole Wheat Bread, (1 cookie, 30g): GI of 60, GL of 9, Net carb= 14g

MEDIUM GLYCEMIC LOAD FOODS A-Z

At DiabeteBalance Diet, we believe in empowering you with a strategic approach to make informed dietary choices for optimal management of diabetes. Our primary focus is on foods with a low glycemic load, which are ideal for maintaining stable blood sugar levels.

However, we understand the importance of variety and occasional indulgences in your diet. Therefore, we also provide comprehensive information on foods falling within the medium glycemic load category. Although not the optimal choice for regular consumption, we believe in giving you a complete understanding of your options to help you navigate your food choices effectively.

For each food item in this medium category, we present key details, including typical serving size, Glycemic Index (GI), Glycemic Load (GL), and Net Carbohydrates. Armed with this information, you can make more conscious decisions, even when deciding to consume these foods on occasion.

It's essential to remember that portion control plays a vital role when indulging in these foods. While occasional consumption is tolerated, we highly recommend reducing the standard serving size to ensure your net carbohydrate intake stays below 15 grams. This approach will help you maintain better blood sugar control while still allowing some flexibility in your diet. By incorporating this balanced approach, you can enjoy occasional treats without compromising your overall diabetes management goals.

▤ Apple Pie, (1 slice, 125g): GI of 40, GL of 18, Net carb= 32g

▤ Apple Turnover, (1 medium, 100g): GI of 45, GL of 15, Net carb= 33g

▤ Bacon Cheddar Biscuits, (1 biscuit, 64g): GI of 62, GL of 12, Net carb= 25g

▤ Bakewell Tart, (1 slice, 80g): GI of 45, GL of 16, Net carb= 35g

▤ Baklava, (1 piece, 33g): GI of 51, GL of 15, Net carb= 29g

▤ Bannock, (1 piece, 60g): GI of 70, GL of 12, Net carb= 24g

▤ Beignets, (1 medium, 60g): GI of 50, GL of 17, Net carb= 34g

▤ Biscuit Sandwiches, (1 sandwich, 130g): GI of 62, GL of 12, Net carb= 28g

▤ Black Forest Cake, (1 slice, 100g): GI of 35, GL of 12, Net carb= 34g

▤ Black Forest Tart, (1 slice, 100g): GI of 65, GL of 16, Net carb= 25g

▤ Blackberry Pie, (1 slice, 125g): GI of 55, GL of 15, Net carb= 29g

▤ Blueberry Custard Tart, (1 slice, 100g): GI of 55, GL of 14, Net carb= 21g

▤ Blueberry Pie, (1 slice, 125g): GI of 60, GL of 17, Net carb= 30g

▤ Boston Cream Pie, (1 slice, 100g): GI of 35, GL of 12, Net carb= 34g

▤ Buttermilk Biscuits, (1 biscuit, 64g): GI of 62, GL of 11, Net carb= 24g

▤ Buttermilk Pie, (1 slice, 125g): GI of 50, GL of 17, Net carb= 38g

▤ Cannoli, (1 medium, 85g): GI of 50, GL of 16, Net carb= 32g

▤ Carrot Cake, (1 slice, 100g): GI of 40, GL of 16, Net carb= 40g

▤ Challah, (1 slice, 40g): GI of 60, GL of 12, Net carb= 20g

▤ Cheesecake, (1 slice, 100g): GI of 35, GL of 10, Net carb= 28g

▤ Chocolate Cake, (1 slice, 100g): GI of 38, GL of 14, Net carb= 35g

▤ Chocolate Chip Biscuits, (1 biscuit, 57g): GI of 62, GL of 14, Net carb= 33g

🍽 Chocolate Chip Cookies, (1 cookie, 30g): GI of 65, GL of 11, Net carb= 19g

🍽 Chocolate Silk Pie, (1 slice, 100g): GI of 65, GL of 19, Net carb= 26g

🍽 Chocolate Tart, (1 slice, 100g): GI of 70, GL of 10, Net carb= 23g

🍽 Churros, (1 medium, 30g): GI of 45, GL of 11, Net carb= 24g

🍽 Ciabatta, (1 serving, 50g): GI of 65, GL of 12, Net carb= 20g

🍽 Cinnamon Roll, (1 small, 60g): GI of 50, GL of 16, Net carb= 31g

🍽 Cinnamon Roll Biscuits, (1 biscuit, 28g): GI of 65, GL of 10, Net carb= 20g

🍽 Coconut Cake, (1 slice, 80g): GI of 70, GL of 18, Net carb= 31g

🍽 Coconut Cream Pie, (1 slice, 100g): GI of 60, GL of 16, Net carb= 26g

🍽 Coffee Cake, (1 slice, 100g): GI of 37, GL of 14, Net carb= 38g

🍽 Cornbread, (1 piece, 60g): GI of 65, GL of 18, Net carb= 28g

🍽 Cornish Pasty, (1 small, 150g): GI of 45, GL of 18, Net carb= 40g

🍽 Croissant, (1 medium,57g): GI of 47, GL of 12, Net carb= 23g

🍽 Custard Tart, (1 slice, 100g): GI of 60, GL of 10, Net carb= 20g

🍽 Dobos Torte, (1 slice, 100g): GI of 35, GL of 11, Net carb= 31g

🍽 Double Chocolate Cookies, (1 cookie, 30g): GI of 70, GL of 13, Net carb= 19g

🍽 Eccles Cake, (1 cake, 60g): GI of 50, GL of 13, Net carb= 27g

🍽 Éclair, (1 medium, 85g): GI of 46, GL of 12, Net carb= 26g

🍽 Empanada, (1 small, 100g): GI of 40, GL of 14, Net carb= 35g

🍽 Focaccia, (1 slice, 50g): GI of 65, GL of 12, Net carb= 20g

▤ Fougasse, (1 serving, 50g): GI of 65, GL of 12, Net carb= 20g

▤ French Bread, (1 slice, 30g): GI of 95, GL of 14, Net carb= 15g

▤ German Chocolate Cake, (1 slice, 100g): GI of 38, GL of 15, Net carb= 38g

▤ Gingerbread Cookies, (1 cookie, 30g): GI of 65, GL of 10, Net carb= 16g

▤ Ham and Cheese Biscuits, (1 biscuit, 60g): GI of 62, GL of 10, Net carb= 20g

▤ Irish Soda Bread, (1 slice, 45g): GI of 65, GL of 13, Net carb= 20g

▤ Italian Bread, (1 slice, 30g): GI of 70, GL of 10, Net carb= 14g

▤ Lemon Cake, (1 slice, 100g): GI of 34, GL of 11, Net carb= 31g

▤ Lemon Meringue Pie, (1 slice, 125g): GI of 45, GL of 17, Net carb= 31g

▤ Lemon Mousse Tart, (1 slice, 100g): GI of 45, GL of 11, Net carb= 22g

▤ Linzer Cookies, (1 cookie, 30g): GI of 55, GL of 10, Net carb= 16g

▤ Marble Cake, (1 slice, 100g): GI of 34, GL of 13, Net carb= 36g

▤ Mille Crepe Cake, (1 slice, 100g): GI of 30, GL of 10, Net carb= 33g

▤ Mixed Berry Pie, (1 slice, 100g): GI of 65, GL of 14, Net carb= 18g

▤ Molasses Cookies, (1 cookie, 30g): GI of 60, GL of 12, Net carb= 17g

▤ Naan, (1 piece, 60g): GI of 62, GL of 16, Net carb= 26g

▤ Oatmeal Raisin Cookies, (1 cookie, 30g): GI of 55, GL of 10, Net carb= 16g

▤ Orange Cake, (1 slice, 80g): GI of 70, GL of 18, Net carb= 31g

▤ Panettone, (1 slice, 50g): GI of 65, GL of 15, Net carb= 23g

▤ Peach Pie, (1 slice, 125g): GI of 50, GL of 16, Net carb= 27g

▤ Pita Bread, (1 small pita, 35g): GI of 57, GL of 10, Net carb= 18g

▤ Pithivier, (1 small, 90g): GI of 50, GL of 18, Net carb= 36g

▤ Pound Cake, (1 slice, 100g): GI of 34, GL of 13, Net carb= 37g

▤ Pretzel, (1 medium, 60g): GI of 75, GL of 16, Net carb= 22g

▤ Puff Pastry, (1 sheet, 79g): GI of 50, GL of 18, Net carb= 36g

▤ Rhubarb Pie, (1 slice, 125g): GI of 50, GL of 14, Net carb= 26g

▤ Simit, (1 piece, 60g): GI of 65, GL of 14, Net carb= 22g

▤ Sponge Cake, (1 slice, 100g): GI of 32, GL of 11, Net carb= 33g

▤ Strawberry Shortcake, (1 slice, 100g): GI of 34, GL of 11, Net carb= 32g

▤ Strawberry Tart, (1 biscuit, 50g): GI of 62, GL of 10, Net carb= 22g

▤ Sugar Cookies, (1 slice, 100g): GI of 45, GL of 17, Net carb= 38g

▤ Sweet Potato Biscuits, (1 cookie, 30g): GI of 65, GL of 10, Net carb= 16g

▤ Tiramisu, (1 small, 60g): GI of 45, GL of 13, Net carb= 28g

▤ Tomato Tart, (1 slice, 100g): GI of 40, GL of 12, Net carb= 30g

▤ Vol-au-vent, (1 slice, 100g): GI of 36, GL of 13, Net carb= 34g

▤ Molasses Cookies, (1 cookie, 30g): GI of 60, GL of 12, Net carb= 17g

▤ Naan, (1 piece, 60g): GI of 62, GL of 16, Net carb= 26g

▤ Oatmeal Raisin Cookies, (1 cookie, 30g): GI of 55, GL of 10, Net carb= 16g

▤ Orange Cake, (1 slice, 80g): GI of 70, GL of 18, Net carb= 31g

▤ Panettone, (1 slice, 50g): GI of 65, GL of 15, Net carb= 23g

Peach Pie, (1 slice, 125g): GI of 50, GL of 16, Net carb= 27g

Pita Bread, (1 small pita, 35g): GI of 57, GL of 10, Net carb= 18g

Pithivier, (1 small, 90g): GI of 50, GL of 18, Net carb= 36g

Pound Cake, (1 slice, 100g): GI of 34, GL of 13, Net carb= 37g

Pretzel, (1 medium, 60g): GI of 75, GL of 16, Net carb= 22g

Puff Pastry, (1 sheet, 79g): GI of 50, GL of 18, Net carb= 36g

Rhubarb Pie, (1 slice, 125g): GI of 50, GL of 14, Net carb= 26g

Simit, (1 piece, 60g): GI of 65, GL of 14, Net carb= 22g

Sponge Cake, (1 slice, 100g): GI of 32, GL of 11, Net carb= 33g

Strawberry Shortcake, (1 slice, 100g): GI of 34, GL of 11, Net carb= 32g

Strawberry Tart, (1 biscuit, 50g): GI of 62, GL of 10, Net carb= 22g

Sugar Cookies, (1 slice, 100g): GI of 45, GL of 17, Net carb= 38g

Sweet Potato Biscuits, (1 cookie, 30g): GI of 65, GL of 10, Net carb= 16g

Tiramisu, (1 small, 60g): GI of 45, GL of 13, Net carb= 28g

Tomato Tart, (1 slice, 100g): GI of 40, GL of 12, Net carb= 30g

Vol-au-vent, (1 slice, 100g): GI of 36, GL of 13, Net carb= 34g

BEVERAGES AND DRINKS

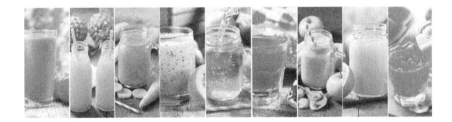

Beverages hold a significant place in our hydration and nourishment routine. For individuals following the DiabeteBalance Diet, grasping the impact of different drinks on glycemic load (GL) and overall health is crucial. This understanding empowers individuals to make informed choices that align with their diabetes management objectives. Below, we delve into the benefits and potential drawbacks of various beverages, offering guidelines for their integration into the DiabeteBalance Diet.

Advantages of Healthy Beverages:

- **Hydration:** Water and similar beverages hydrate without affecting blood glucose levels.

- **Nutrient-Rich Options:** Drinks such as vegetable juice, fortified plant-based milk, and low-fat dairy products provide vital nutrients. This aids in overall health and combats deficiencies often seen in Type 2 Diabetes (T2D).
- **Convenient Protein Source:** Protein powders mixed with water or milk are a handy protein source with minimal impact on blood glucose levels.

Drawbacks of Certain Beverages:

- **High Sugar Content:** Many commercial drinks, including sodas and sweetened coffees, have excessive added sugars. This can spike blood sugar levels and hinder weight loss and diabetes management.
- **Lack of Fiber:** Most beverages do not contain dietary fiber, vital for stable blood sugar levels and fullness.
- **Artificial Sweeteners:** Some "diet" drinks may have potential adverse health effects and can lead to cravings for sweets.

Guidelines for Incorporating Beverages into the DiabeteBalance Diet:

- **Prioritize Water:** With a GL of zero, water is the optimal hydration choice.
- **Opt for Unsweetened Drinks:** Choose unsweetened beverages or add a slice of citrus or cucumber for a low-calorie flavor boost.
- **Limit Fruit Juices:** Due to high sugar content, limit or dilute fruit juices.
- **Monitor Dairy Consumption:** While low-fat dairy provides essential nutrients, it also contains lactose. Mind the portion sizes.
- **Avoid Sugary and Artificially Sweetened Drinks:** Steer clear of high-sugar and artificially sweetened drinks, as they can have negative health implications.

- **Utilize Protein Powders:** Unsweetened protein powders can be a convenient, low-GL protein source.
- **Practice Portion Control:** Even healthy drinks can lead to high-calorie intake if overconsumed. Review the provided list for details on GL, GI, and net carb content per typical serving size (15-20 grams).

Comprehensive Selection for the DiabeteBalance Diet:

The following list aligns with the DiabeteBalance Diet, offering details on serving size, Glycemic Index (GI), Glycemic Load (GL), and Net Carbohydrates. This data helps guide portion control and effective meal planning, with entries organized alphabetically for ease of reference.

LOW GLYCEMIC LOAD FOODS A-Z

📃 Almond Milk, (1 cup (240ml)): GI of 30, GL of 0.6, Net carb= 2g

📃 Almond Milk, unsweetened, (1 cup (240ml)): GI of 30, GL of 0.3, Net carb= 1g

📃 Almond-Flavored Water, (1 cup (240ml)): GI of 0, GL of 0, Net carb= 0g

📃 Americano, (1 cup (240ml)): GI of 0, GL of 0, Net carb= 0g

📃 Apple Cider Vinegar (diluted as a beverage), (1 cup (240ml)): GI of 0, GL of 0, Net carb= 0g

📃 Basil Infused Water, (1 cup (240ml)): GI of 0, GL of 0, Net carb= 0g

📃 Beer, (1 cup (240ml)): GI of 50, GL of 4, Net carb= 8g

📃 Beer (light), (1 cup (240ml)): GI of 50, GL of 2, Net carb= 4g

📃 Beer (regular), (1 cup (240ml)): GI of 50, GL of 4, Net carb= 8g

⊞ Beet Kvass, (1 cup (240ml)): GI of 60, GL of 6, Net carb= 10g

⊞ Black Tea, (1 cup (240ml)): GI of 0, GL of 0, Net carb= 0g

⊞ Bloody Mary, (1 cup (240ml)): GI of 0, GL of 0, Net carb= 6g

⊞ Blueberry Infused Water, (1 cup (240ml)): GI of 0, GL of 0, Net carb= 0g

⊞ Bulletproof Coffee, (1 cup (240ml)): GI of 0, GL of 0, Net carb= 0g

⊞ Bulletproof Coffee (with MCT oil), (1 cup (240ml)): GI of 0, GL of 0, Net carb= 0g

⊞ Buttermilk, (1 cup (240ml)): GI of 30, GL of 3.3, Net carb= 11g

⊞ Café au lait, (1 cup (240ml)): GI of 30, GL of 1.2, Net carb= 4g

⊞ Caffè Breve, (1 cup (240ml)): GI of 50, GL of 2, Net carb= 4g

⊞ Caffè Corretto, (1 cup (240ml)): GI of 0, GL of 0, Net carb= 0g

⊞ Cappuccino, (1 cup (240ml)): GI of 50, GL of 4, Net carb= 8g

⊞ Carbonated Water with Natural Flavors, (1 cup (240ml)): GI of 0, GL of 0, Net carb= 0g

⊞ Carbonated Water with Stevia and Natural Flavors, (1 cup (240ml)): GI of 0, GL of 0, Net carb= 0g

⊞ Cashew Milk, (1 cup (240ml)): GI of 30, GL of 1.2, Net carb= 4g

⊞ Cashew Milk, unsweetened, (1 cup (240ml)): GI of 35, GL of 0.7, Net carb= 2g

⊞ Chai Tea, (1 cup (240ml)): GI of 0, GL of 0, Net carb= 0g

⊞ Chamomile Tea, (1 cup (240ml)): GI of 0, GL of 0, Net carb= 0g

⊞ Cherry Infused Water, (1 cup (240ml)): GI of 0, GL of 0, Net carb= 0g

⊞ Citrus Infused Water, (1 cup (240ml)): GI of 0, GL of 0, Net carb= 0g

⊟ Club Soda, (1 cup (240ml)): GI of 0, GL of 0, Net carb= 0g

⊟ Coconut Milk, (1 cup (240ml)): GI of 45, GL of 2.7, Net carb= 6g

⊟ Coconut Milk Kefir, (1 cup (240ml)): GI of 30, GL of 1.2, Net carb= 4g

⊟ Coconut Milk, unsweetened, (1 cup (240ml)): GI of 45, GL of 0.9, Net carb= 2g

⊟ Coconut Water, (1 cup (240ml)): GI of 35, GL of 3.2, Net carb= 9g

⊟ Coconut Water Kefir, (1 cup (240ml)): GI of 40, GL of 2.4, Net carb= 6g

⊟ Coconut-Flavored Water, (1 cup (240ml)): GI of 0, GL of 0, Net carb= 0g

⊟ Cold Brew Coffee, (1 cup (240ml)): GI of 0, GL of 0, Net carb= 0g

⊟ Cortado, (4 fl oz (120g)): GI of 0, GL of 0, Net carb= 0g

⊟ Cucumber Infused Water, (1 cup (240ml)): GI of 0, GL of 0, Net carb= 0g

⊟ Diet Cola, (1 cup (240ml)): GI of 0, GL of 0, Net carb= 0g

⊟ Diet Lemon-Lime Soda, (1 cup (240ml)): GI of 0, GL of 0, Net carb= 0g

⊟ Diet Root Beer, (1 cup (240ml)): GI of 0, GL of 0, Net carb= 0g

⊟ Doppio, (¼ cup (60ml)): GI of 0, GL of 0, Net carb= 0g

⊟ Electrolyte Water, (1 cup (240ml)): GI of 0, GL of 0, Net carb= 0g

⊟ Energy Drink (sugar-free), (1 cup (240ml)): GI of 0, GL of 0, Net carb= 0g

⊟ Erythritol-Sweetened Soda, (1 cup (240ml)): GI of 0, GL of 0, Net carb= 0g

⊟ Espresso, (¼ cup (60ml)): GI of 0, GL of 0, Net carb= 0g

▤ Flat White, (1 cup (240ml)): GI of 0, GL of 0, Net carb= 0g

▤ Flavored Tea, (1 cup (240ml)): GI of 0, GL of 0, Net carb= 0g

▤ Flax Milk, (1 cup (240ml)): GI of 45, GL of 0.9, Net carb= 2g

▤ Flax Milk, unsweetened, (1 cup (240ml)): GI of 45, GL of 0.5, Net carb= 1g

▤ Fruit Kefir, (1 cup (240ml)): GI of 30, GL of 2.7, Net carb= 9g

▤ Fruit Wine, (5 fl oz (148g)): GI of 30, GL of 2.7, Net carb= 9g

▤ Ginger Tea, (1 cup (240ml)): GI of 0, GL of 0, Net carb= 0g

▤ Green Tea, (1 cup (240ml)): GI of 0, GL of 0, Net carb= 0g

▤ Green Tea-Flavored Water, (1 cup (240ml)): GI of 0, GL of 0, Net carb= 0g

▤ Hazelnut Milk, (1 cup (240ml)): GI of 30, GL of 1.2, Net carb= 4g

▤ Hazelnut Milk, unsweetened, (1 cup (240ml)): GI of 30, GL of 0.6, Net carb= 2g

▤ Hemp Milk, (1 cup (240ml)): GI of 30, GL of 0.6, Net carb= 2g

▤ Hemp Milk, unsweetened, (1 cup (240ml)): GI of 30, GL of 0.3, Net carb= 1g

▤ Herbal Fermented Teas, (1 cup (240ml)): GI of 0, GL of 0, Net carb= 0g

▤ Herbal Infusion (e.g., Chamomile), (1 cup (240ml)): GI of 0, GL of 0, Net carb= 0g

▤ Herbal Tea, (1 cup (240ml)): GI of 0, GL of 0, Net carb= 0g

▤ Herbal-Infused Water (like rosemary or lavender), (1 cup (240ml)): GI of 0, GL of 0, Net carb= 0g

▤ Hot Apple Toddy, (1 cup (240ml)): GI of 0, GL of 0, Net carb= 10g

▤ Hot Coconut Milk with Cinnamon and Turmeric, (1 cup (240ml)): GI of 0, GL of 0, Net carb= 0g

▤ Hot Lemon Water, (1 cup (240ml)): GI of 0, GL of 0, Net carb= 0g

▤ Hot Tea, (1 cup (240ml)): GI of 0, GL of 0, Net carb= 0g

▤ Iced Coffee, (1 cup (240ml)): GI of 0, GL of 0, Net carb= 0g

▤ Iced Coffee with Milk, (1 cup (240ml)): GI of 0, GL of 0, Net carb= 0g

▤ Iced Matcha Green Tea Latte, (1 cup (240ml)): GI of 0, GL of 0, Net carb= 0g

▤ Iced Tea, (1 cup (240ml)): GI of 0, GL of 0, Net carb= 0g

▤ Isotonic Beverage, (1 cup (240ml)): GI of 50, GL of 5, Net carb= 10g

▤ Jun Tea, (1 cup (240ml)): GI of 20, GL of 1, Net carb= 5g

▤ Kefir, (1 cup (240ml)): GI of 30, GL of 1.2, Net carb= 4g

▤ Kiwi Infused Water, (1 cup (240ml)): GI of 0, GL of 0, Net carb= 0g

▤ Kombucha, (1 cup (240ml)): GI of 10, GL of 0.2, Net carb= 2g

▤ Kvass, (1 cup (240ml)): GI of 40, GL of 3, Net carb= 7g

▤ Laban Ayran, (1 cup (240ml)): GI of 30, GL of 1.2, Net carb= 4g

▤ Lactose-Free Protein Drink, (1 cup (240ml)): GI of 30, GL of 0.9, Net carb= 3g

▤ Lassi Low-carb Drink, (1 cup (240ml)): GI of 30, GL of 3, Net carb= 10g

▤ Latte, (1 cup (240ml)): GI of 40, GL of 4, Net carb= 10g

▤ Latte Macchiato, (1 cup (240ml)): GI of 40, GL of 4, Net carb= 10g

▤ Lemon Infused Water, (1 cup (240ml)): GI of 0, GL of 0, Net carb= 0g

▤ Low-Calorie Energy Drink, (1 cup (240ml)): GI of 0, GL of 0, Net carb= 0g

▤ Low-Calorie Fruit-Flavored Carbonated Drink, (1 cup (240ml)): GI of 50, GL of 5, Net carb= 10g

▤ Low-Calorie Tonic Water, (1 cup (240ml)): GI of 50, GL of 5, Net carb= 10g

▤ Macadamia Milk, (1 cup (240ml)): GI of 35, GL of 1.1, Net carb= 3g

▤ Macadamia Milk, unsweetened, (1 cup (240ml)): GI of 35, GL of 0.7, Net carb= 2g

▤ Macchiato, (1 cup (240ml)): GI of 40, GL of 4, Net carb= 10g

▤ Mango-Flavored Water, (1 cup (240ml)): GI of 0, GL of 0, Net carb= 0g

▤ Margarita, (1 cup (240ml)): GI of 0, GL of 0, Net carb= 0g

▤ Masala Chai, (1 cup (240ml)): GI of 30, GL of 3, Net carb= 10g

▤ Matcha Latte, (1 cup (240ml)): GI of 0, GL of 0, Net carb= 0g

▤ Matcha Tea, (1 cup (240ml)): GI of 0, GL of 0, Net carb= 0g

▤ Mead, (1 cup (240ml)): GI of 10, GL of 2, Net carb= 20g

▤ Milk (2%), (1 cup (240ml)): GI of 30, GL of 3.6, Net carb= 12g

▤ Milk (skimmed), (1 cup (240ml)): GI of 30, GL of 3.6, Net carb= 12g

▤ Milk (whole), (1 cup (240ml)): GI of 30, GL of 3.6, Net carb= 12g

▤ Milk Kefir, (1 cup (240ml)): GI of 30, GL of 1.2, Net carb= 4g

▤ Mint and Lime-Flavored Water, (1 cup (240ml)): GI of 0, GL of 0, Net carb= 0g

▤ Mint Infused Water, (1 cup (240ml)): GI of 0, GL of 0, Net carb= 0g

▤ Mint Tea, (1 cup (240ml)): GI of 0, GL of 0, Net carb= 0g

▤ Monk Fruit unsweetened Soda, (1 cup (240ml)): GI of 0, GL of 0, Net carb= 0g

▤ Moroccan Mint Tea, Unsweetened, (1 cup (240ml)): GI of 0, GL of 0, Net carb= 0g

▤ Mulled Wine, (5 fl oz (148g)): GI of 50, GL of 7.5, Net carb= 15g

▤ Oolong Tea, (1 cup (240ml)): GI of 0, GL of 0, Net carb= 0g

▤ Pea Protein Milk, (1 cup (240ml)): GI of 30, GL of 0.6, Net carb= 2g

▤ Pea Protein Milk, sweetened, (1 cup (240ml)): GI of 30, GL of 4.2, Net carb= 14g

▤ Pea Protein Milk, unsweetened, (1 cup (240ml)): GI of 30, GL of 0.3, Net carb= 1g

▤ Peach-Flavored Water, (1 cup (240ml)): GI of 0, GL of 0, Net carb= 0g

▤ Pineapple Infused Water, (1 cup (240ml)): GI of 0, GL of 0, Net carb= 0g

▤ Pistachio Milk, (1 cup (240ml)): GI of 35, GL of 1.8, Net carb= 5g

▤ Pistachio Milk, sweetened, (1 cup (240ml)): GI of 60, GL of 9, Net carb= 15g

▤ Pistachio Milk, unsweetened, (1 cup (240ml)): GI of 25, GL of 0.8, Net carb= 3g

▤ Pomegranate Infused Water, (1 cup (240ml)): GI of 0, GL of 0, Net carb= 0g

▤ Protein Shake, (1 cup (240ml)): GI of 25, GL of 1.3, Net carb= 5g

▤ Protein Shake (Whey Based), (1 cup (240ml)): GI of 30, GL of 2.1, Net carb= 7g

▤ Quinoa Milk, (1 cup (240ml)): GI of 35, GL of 1.8, Net carb= 5g

▤ Quinoa Milk, unsweetened, (1 cup (240ml)): GI of 25, GL of 0.8, Net carb= 3g

▤ Raspberry Infused Water, (1 cup (240ml)): GI of 0, GL of 0, Net carb= 0g

▤ Rice Wine, (5 fl oz (100g)): GI of 10, GL of 0.3, Net carb= 3g

▤ Ristretto, (1 fl oz (30g)): GI of 0, GL of 0, Net carb= 0g

▤ Rooibos Tea, (1 cup (240ml)): GI of 0, GL of 0, Net carb= 0g

▤ Rum, (1 fl oz (30g)): GI of 0, GL of 0, Net carb= 0g

▤ Sake, (5 fl oz (100g)): GI of 20, GL of 0.2, Net carb= 1g

▤ Seltzer Water, (1 cup (240ml)): GI of 0, GL of 0, Net carb= 0g

▤ Shrub (drinking vinegar), (1 cup (240ml)): GI of 0, GL of 0, Net carb= 0g

▤ Soy Milk, (1 cup (240ml)): GI of 30, GL of 2.4, Net carb= 8g

▤ Soy Milk, unsweetened, (1 cup (240ml)): GI of 20, GL of 0.8, Net carb= 4g

▤ Sparkling Iced Tea (unsweetened), (1 cup (240ml)): GI of 0, GL of 0, Net carb= 0g

▤ Sparkling Water, (1 cup (240ml)): GI of 0, GL of 0, Net carb= 0g

▤ Sports Drink (low-carb), (1 cup (240ml)): GI of 0, GL of 0, Net carb= 0g

▤ Stevia-Sweetened Soda, (1 cup (240ml)): GI of 0, GL of 0, Net carb= 0g

▤ Strawberry Infused Water, (1 cup (240ml)): GI of 0, GL of 0, Net carb= 0g

▤ Sugar-Free Cream Soda, (1 cup (240ml)): GI of 0, GL of 0, Net carb= 0g

▤ Sugar-Free Energy Drink, (1 cup (240ml)): GI of 0, GL of 0, Net carb= 0g

▤ Sugar-Free Tonic Water, (1 cup (240ml)): GI of 0, GL of 0, Net carb= 0g

▤ Switchel, (1 cup (240ml)): GI of 25, GL of 2.5, Net carb= 10g

▤ Tequila, (1 fl oz (30g)): GI of 0, GL of 0, Net carb= 0g

▤ Tiger Nut Milk, (1 cup (240ml)): GI of 45, GL of 3.6, Net carb= 8g

▤ Tiger Nut Milk, unsweetened, (1 cup (240ml)): GI of 30, GL of 0.3, Net carb= 1g

▤ Turmeric Latte, (1 cup (240ml)): GI of 40, GL of 5.6, Net carb= 14g

▤ Turmeric Tea, (1 cup (240ml)): GI of 0, GL of 0, Net carb= 0g

▤ Vanilla-Flavored Water, (1 cup (240ml)): GI of 0, GL of 0, Net carb= 0g

▤ Vienna Coffee, (1 cup (240ml)): GI of 0, GL of 0, Net carb= 0g

▤ Vinegar (diluted as a beverage), (1 cup (240ml)): GI of 0, GL of 0, Net carb= 0g

▤ Vitamin-Enriched Water, (1 cup (240ml)): GI of 0, GL of 0, Net carb= 0g

▤ Vodka, (1 fl oz (30g)): GI of 0, GL of 0, Net carb= 0g

▤ Walnut Milk, unsweetened, (1 cup (240ml)): GI of 25, GL of 0.3, Net carb= 1g

▤ Water Kefir, (1 cup (240ml)): GI of 30, GL of 1.5, Net carb= 5g

▤ Water with Natural Fruit Flavors, (1 cup (240ml)): GI of 0, GL of 0, Net carb= 0g

▤ Whiskey, (1 fl oz (30g)): GI of 0, GL of 0, Net carb= 0g

▤ White Tea, (1 cup (240ml)): GI of 0, GL of 0, Net carb= 0g

▤ Wine, (5 fl oz (148g)): GI of 0, GL of 0, Net carb= 0g

▤ Wine (red), (5 fl oz (148g)): GI of 0, GL of 0, Net carb= 0g

▤ Wine (white), (5 fl oz (148g)): GI of 0, GL of 0, Net carb= 0g

▤ Yakult, (2.7 fl oz (80g)): GI of 50, GL of 6, Net carb= 12g

▤ Zero Calorie Energy Drink, (1 cup (240ml)): GI of 0, GL of 0, Net carb= 0g

▤ Zero Sugar Cola, (1 cup (240ml)): GI of 0, GL of 0, Net carb= 0g

▤ Zero Sugar Ginger Ale, (1 cup (240ml)): GI of 0, GL of 0, Net carb= 0g

---

MEDIUM GLYCEMIC LOAD FOODS A-Z

In the DiabeteBalance Diet, we prioritize a strategic approach that empowers you to make informed dietary choices. While we emphasize foods with a low glycemic load as the adequate choice for optimally managing diabetes, we understand the need for variety and occasional indulgences.

Thus, we also provide comprehensive information on foods that fall within the medium glycemic load category. These are not the optimal option for regular consumption, but we believe in giving you a complete understanding of your options to help you navigate your food choices.

For each food item in this medium category, we present key details including typical serving size, Glycemic Index (GI), Glycemic Load (GL), and Net Carbohydrates. Armed with this information, you can make more conscious decisions even when you decide to consume these foods on occasion.

However, it's crucial to remember that portion control is vital when indulging in these foods. While they can be tolerated occasionally, we highly recommend reducing the standard serving size to ensure that your intake stays below 15 grams of net carbohydrates. This approach will help you maintain better blood sugar control while still allowing some flexibility in your diet.

▤ Caffè Mocha, (1 cup (240ml)): GI of 50, GL of 16, Net carb= 32g

▤ Caramel Latte, (1 cup (240ml)): GI of 50, GL of 12.5, Net carb= 25g

▤ Caramel Macchiato, (1 cup (240ml)): GI of 50, GL of 12.5, Net carb= 25g

▤ Chocolate Milk, (1 cup (240ml)): GI of 60, GL of 13.8, Net carb= 23g

▤ Coconut Milk, sweetened, (1 cup (240ml)): GI of 50, GL of 10.5, Net carb= 21g

▤ Hot Mocha, (1 cup (240ml)): GI of 50, GL of 15, Net carb= 30g

▤ Hot Peppermint Mocha, (1 cup (240ml)): GI of 50, GL of 15, Net carb= 30g

▤ Iced Chai Tea Latte, (1 cup (240ml)): GI of 50, GL of 12.5, Net carb= 25g

▤ Malt Drink, (1 cup (240ml)): GI of 50, GL of 17.5, Net carb= 35g

▤ Oat Milk, (1 cup (240ml)): GI of 69, GL of 16.6, Net carb= 24g

▤ Post-workout Recovery Drink, (1 cup (240ml)): GI of 50, GL of 12.5, Net carb= 25g

▤ Pre-workout Energy Drink, (1 cup (240ml)): GI of 65, GL of 19.5, Net carb= 30g

▤ Rice Milk, unsweetened, (1 cup (240ml)): GI of 75, GL of 11.3, Net carb= 15g

■ Sarsaparilla, (1 cup (240ml)): GI of 50, GL of 12.5, Net carb= 25g

■ Sports Drinks, (1 cup (240ml)): GI of 60, GL of 18, Net carb= 30g

■ Tepache, (1 cup (240ml)): GI of 55, GL of 13.8, Net carb= 25g

■ Thai Iced Tea, (1 cup (240ml)): GI of 50, GL of 12.5, Net carb= 25g

■ Tiger Nut Milk, sweetened, (1 cup (240ml)): GI of 65, GL of 15.6, Net carb= 24g

■ Tonic Water, (1 cup (240ml)): GI of 50, GL of 12.5, Net carb= 25g

■ Yogurt Smoothie, (1 cup (240ml)): GI of 50, GL of 15, Net carb= 30g

BEEF, VEAL, PORK, LAMB AND POULTRY

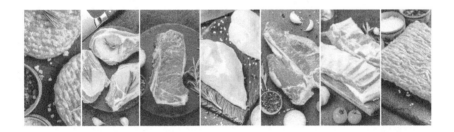

Meat products, when chosen with care and consumed in moderation, can be an integral part of the DiabeteBalance Diet. Analyzing their glycemic load (GL), nutritional content, and understanding the pros and cons of meat consumption will assist individuals in making dietary choices that align with diabetes management and overall well-being.

Benefits of Meat in the DiabeteBalance Diet:

- **Nutrient Density:** Meat is rich in essential nutrients like iron, zinc, and B vitamins, aiding overall health and warding off deficiencies common in diabetes.
- **Complete Protein Source:** Meat serves as a complete protein

source, supplying all nine vital amino acids required for muscle development, recovery, and general well-being. Especially, lean meats are advantageous for those with type 2 diabetes, ensuring they achieve sufficient protein consumption.

Potential Drawbacks of Meat:

- **Saturated Fats:** Certain meats, particularly fatty and processed variants, are high in saturated fats. Excess consumption may lead to weight gain and heart disease risks, which are detrimental for type 2 diabetes management.
- **Processed Meats:** Meats like sausages and bacon often contain unhealthy levels of sodium, nitrates, and additives, making them incompatible with the DiabeteBalance Diet.

Guidelines for Incorporating Meat into the DiabeteBalance Diet:

- **Opt for Lean Meats:** Prefer lean cuts of red meat, skinless poultry, and fish to minimize saturated fat and calorie intake.
- **Avoid Highly Processed Meats:** Such meats are often rich in sodium and unhealthy fats and should be avoided.
- **Healthy Cooking Methods:** Utilize methods like grilling, baking, or steaming instead of frying to minimize unhealthy fats.
- **Serving Size and Nutritional Information:** Follow the tailored serving sizes and nutritional guidelines provided in the lists of this chapter. They focus on meats that are compatible with the DiabeteBalance Diet and exclude high-sodium and overly processed variants.

Comprehensive Selection for the DiabeteBalance Diet:

Below, you'll find an alphabetical list of meats that fully comply with the DiabeteBalance Diet. Details on serving size, Glycemic Index (GI), Glycemic Load (GL), and Net Carbohydrates are included. This information guides you in making well-informed decisions on portion sizes and meal planning.

▤ Bacon, Uncured, low-sodium, no added sugar Grilled or Baked, (3 slices, 35g): GI of 0, GL of 0, Net carb= 0g

▤ Beef Brisket, Oven-Roasted, (3 oz, 85g): GI of 0, GL of 0, Net carb= 0g

▤ Beef Brisket, Slow-Cooked, (3 oz, 85g): GI of 0, GL of 0, Net carb= 0g

▤ Beef Burger, lean, Broiled, (1 burger, 150g): GI of 0, GL of 0, Net carb= 0g

▤ Beef Burger, lean, Grilled, (1 burger, 150g): GI of 0, GL of 0, Net carb= 0g

▤ Beef jerky, low-sodium, (1 oz, 28g): GI of 0-5, GL of 0, Net carb= 3g

▤ Beef Ribs, Slow-Cooked, (3 ribs, 180g): GI of 0, GL of 0, Net carb= 0g

▤ Beef Roast, Marinated and Oven-Roasted, (4 oz, 113g): GI of 0, GL of 0, Net carb= 0g

▤ Beef Roast, Oven-Roasted, (4 oz, 113g): GI of 0, GL of 0, Net carb= 0g

▤ Beef Roast, Slow-Cooked, (4 oz, 113g): GI of 0, GL of 0, Net carb= 0g

▤ Beef Roast, Slow-Cooked with Vegetables, (4 oz, 113g): GI of 0, GL of 0, Net carb= 1g

▤ Beef Sirloin, Broiled, (4 oz, 113g): GI of 0, GL of 0, Net carb= 0g

▦ Beef Sirloin, Grilled, (4 oz, 113g): GI of 0, GL of 0, Net carb= 0g

▦ Beef Sirloin, Marinated and Pan-Seared, (4 oz, 113g): GI of 25-35, GL of 3, Net carb= 10g

▦ Beef Sirloin, Pan-Seared, (4 oz, 113g): GI of 0, GL of 0, Net carb= 0g

▦ Beef Steak, Grilled, (4 oz, 113g): GI of 0, GL of 0, Net carb= 0g

▦ Beef Steak, Marinated and Grilled, (4 oz, 113g): GI of 25-35, GL of 2, Net carb= 5g

▦ Beef Steak, Marinated and Pan-Fried, (4 oz, 113g): GI of 30-35, GL of 2, Net carb= 5g

▦ Beef Steak, Oven-Baked, (4 oz, 113g): GI of 0, GL of 0, Net carb= 0g

▦ Beef Steak, Pan-Seared, (4 oz, 113g): GI of 0, GL of 0, Net carb= 0g

▦ Beef Stew, Slow-Cooked, (1 cup, 240g): GI of 0, GL of 0, Net carb= 0g

▦ Beef Stew, with Carrots and Peas, (1 cup, 240g): GI of 0, GL of 0, Net carb= 5g

▦ Beef Stew, with Corn and Green Beans, (1 cup, 240g): GI of 15-25, GL of 1, Net carb= 5g

▦ Beef Stew, with Mushrooms, (1 cup, 240g): GI of 15-25, GL of 1, Net carb= 5g

▦ Beef sticks, low-sodium, (1 oz, 28g): GI of 0, GL of 0, Net carb= 1g

▦ Beef Stir-Fry, with Vegetables, (1 cup, 200g): GI of 0, GL of 0, Net carb= 0g

▦ Bison Burger, Grilled, (1 patty): GI of 0, GL of 0, Net carb= 0g

▦ Bison Steak, Grilled, (3 oz): GI of 0, GL of 0, Net carb= 0g

▦ Chicken Breast, Grilled, (4 oz, 113g): GI of 0, GL of 0, Net carb= 0g

▤ Chicken Breast, Marinated and Baked, (4 oz, 113g): GI of 25-35, GL of 2, Net carb= 5g

▤ Chicken Breast, Marinated and Grilled, (4 oz, 113g): GI of 0-5, GL of 0, Net carb= 5g

▤ Chicken Breast, Pan-Seared, (4 oz, 113g): GI of 0, GL of 0, Net carb= 0g

▤ Chicken Cutlet, Grilled, (1 cutlet, 120g): GI of 20-30, GL of 1, Net carb= 5g

▤ Chicken Drumstick, Baked, (1 drumstick, 85g): GI of 0, GL of 0, Net carb= 0g

▤ Chicken Drumstick, Roasted, (1 drumstick, 85g): GI of 0, GL of 0, Net carb= 0g

▤ Chicken Tender, Baked, (4 tenders, 85g): GI of 40-55, GL of 3, Net carb= 5g

▤ Chicken Thigh, Baked, (1 thigh, 120g): GI of 0, GL of 0, Net carb= 0g

▤ Chicken Thigh, Grilled, (1 thigh, 120g): GI of 0, GL of 0, Net carb= 0g

▤ Chuck roast, Grilled or Broiled, (3 oz, 85g): GI of 0, GL of 0, Net carb= 0g

▤ Cornish Game Hen, Roasted, (1 hen): GI of 0, GL of 0, Net carb= 0g

▤ Duck Breast, Pan-Seared, (3 oz): GI of 0, GL of 0, Net carb= 0g

▤ Duck Leg, Roasted, (1 leg): GI of 0, GL of 0, Net carb= 0g

▤ Elk Steak, Grilled, (3 oz): GI of 0, GL of 0, Net carb= 0g

▤ Filet mignon, Grilled or Broiled, (3 oz, 85g): GI of 0, GL of 0, Net carb= 0g

▤ Flank steak, Grilled or Broiled, (3 oz, 85g): GI of 0, GL of 0, Net carb= 0g

▤ Goose, Roasted, (3 oz): GI of 0, GL of 0, Net carb= 0g

▤ Ground Beef, , Lean, low-sodium, homemade, Baked, (3 oz, 85g): GI of 0, GL of 0, Net carb= 0g

▤ Ground Beef, lean, low-sodium, Broiled, (3 oz, 85g): GI of 0, GL of 0, Net carb= 0g

▤ Ground Beef, lean, Lean, low-sodium, homemade, Grilled, (3 oz, 85g): GI of 0, GL of 0, Net carb= 0g

▤ Ground Beef, Lean, low-sodium, homemade, Pan-Fried, (3 oz, 85g): GI of 0, GL of 0, Net carb= 0g

▤ Ground Lamb, lean, low-sodium, Pan-Fried, (3 oz): GI of 0, GL of 0, Net carb= 0g

▤ Ground meat products, Lean, homemade Grilled or Broiled, (3 oz, 85g): GI of 0, GL of 0, Net carb= 0g

▤ Ground Pork, Pan-Fried, (3 oz, 85g): GI of 40-55, GL of 2, Net carb= 5g

▤ Ground Turkey, Baked, (3 oz): GI of 0, GL of 0, Net carb= 0g

▤ Ground Turkey, Pan-Fried, (3 oz): GI of 0, GL of 0, Net carb= 0g

▤ Lamb Chops, Grilled, (3 oz): GI of 0, GL of 0, Net carb= 0g

▤ Lamb Roast, Oven-Roasted, (3 oz): GI of 0, GL of 0, Net carb= 0g

▤ Lamb Shank, Braised, (3 oz): GI of 0, GL of 0, Net carb= 0g

▤ Ostrich Steak, Grilled, (3 oz): GI of 0, GL of 0, Net carb= 0g

▤ Pork Belly, Braised, (3 oz, 85g): GI of 20-30, GL of 2, Net carb= 5g

▤ Pork Belly, Roasted, (3 oz, 85g): GI of 35-50, GL of 3, Net carb= 5g

▤ Pork Loin Chop, Grilled, (1 chop, 150g): GI of 20-30, GL of 3, Net carb= 5g

▤ Pork Loin Roast, Oven-Roasted, (3 oz, 85g): GI of 30-45, GL of 2, Net carb= 5g

▤ Pork Loin Roast, Slow-Cooked, (4 oz, 113g): GI of 25-35, GL of 2, Net carb= 5g

▤ Pork Loin, Oven-Baked, (4 oz, 113g): GI of 30-45, GL of 1, Net carb= 5g

▤ Pork Ribs, Slow-Cooked, (3 ribs, 180g): GI of 25-35, GL of 3, Net carb= 5g

▤ Pork Roast, Oven-Roasted, (4 oz, 113g): GI of 35-50, GL of 3, Net carb= 5g

▤ Pork Shoulder, Slow-Roasted, (3 oz, 85g): GI of 50-65, GL of 3, Net carb= 5g

▤ Pork Tenderloin, Marinated and Grilled, (4 oz, 113g): GI of 25-35, GL of 2, Net carb= 5g

▤ Quail, Grilled or Roasted, (1 quail): GI of 0, GL of 0, Net carb= 0g

▤ Rabbit, Braised or Grilled, (3 oz): GI of 0, GL of 0, Net carb= 0g

▤ Ribeye steak, Grilled or Broiled, (3 oz, 85g): GI of 0, GL of 0, Net carb= 0g

▤ Round steak, Grilled or Broiled, (3 oz, 85g): GI of 0, GL of 0, Net carb= 0g

▤ Sausage, Lean, Low-sodium, Grilled or Baked, (3 oz, 85g): GI of 0, GL of 0, Net carb= 1g

▤ Short ribs, Grilled or Broiled, (3 oz, 85g): GI of 0, GL of 0, Net carb= 0g

▤ Sirloin steak, Grilled or Broiled, (3 oz, 85g): GI of 0, GL of 0, Net carb= 0g

▤ Skirt steak, Grilled or Broiled, (3 oz, 85g): GI of 0, GL of 0, Net carb= 0g

▤ T-bone steak, Grilled or Broiled, (3 oz, 85g): GI of 0, GL of 0, Net carb= 0g

▤ Tri-tip, Grilled or Broiled, (3 oz, 85g): GI of 0, GL of 0, Net carb= 0g

▤ Turkey Breast, Roasted, (3 oz): GI of 0, GL of 0, Net carb= 0g

▤ Turkey Burger, lean, low-sodium, homemade, Grilled, (1 patty): GI of 0, GL of 0, Net carb= 0g

▤ Turkey Drumstick, Roasted, (1 drumstick): GI of 0, GL of 0, Net carb= 0g

▤ Turkey Tender, Baked, (3 oz): GI of 0, GL of 0, Net carb= 0g

▤ Turkey Thigh, Roasted, (1 thigh): GI of 0, GL of 0, Net carb= 0g

▤ Turkey Wing, Baked, (1 wing): GI of 0, GL of 0, Net carb= 0g

▤ Veal Roast, Oven-Roasted, (3 oz): GI of 0, GL of 0, Net carb= 0g

▤ Veal Scallopini, Pan-Seared, (3 oz): GI of 0, GL of 0, Net carb= 0g

▤ Venison Steak, Grilled, (3 oz): GI of 0, GL of 0, Net carb= 0g

▤ Veal Roast, Oven-Roasted, (3 oz): GI of 0, GL of 0, Net carb= 0g

▤ Veal Scallopini, Pan-Seared, (3 oz): GI of 0, GL of 0, Net carb= 0g

DAIRY AND PLANT-BASED ALTERNATIVES

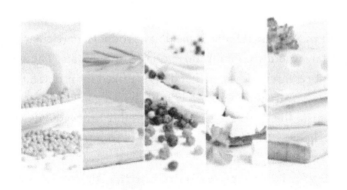

Dairy products are prevalent in numerous diets, including those tailored for better management of diabetes. Knowing how to include dairy while being mindful of its glycemic load (GL) and alignment with the principles of the DiabeteBalance Diet is essential. Below, we delve into the advantages and potential considerations of dairy, along with guidelines for incorporating it into a diabetes-friendly diet.

Benefits of Dairy:

- **Rich in Nutrients:** Dairy products such as cheese are dense in essential nutrients like calcium, protein, and vitamin D. For instance, a 1 oz (28 grams) serving of cheese fits well within the DiabeteBalance Diet, providing vital support to overall health.
- **Source of Probiotics:** Fermented dairy like yogurt, kefir and cottage cheese offers probiotics, beneficial bacteria that may help with glycemic control and gut health.

Drawbacks of Dairy:

- **Lactose Content:** The lactose in dairy can elevate blood glucose levels, and lactose intolerance may limit consumption.
- **High in Saturated Fats:** Some dairy products, particularly full-fat varieties, contain substantial saturated fats. Though recent research indicates that dairy-derived saturated fats may be less harmful, moderation is still advised.
- **Potential for Processed Products:** Highly processed dairy can contain excessive added sugars and sodium.

Guidelines for Incorporating Dairy into the DiabeteBalance Diet:

- **Opt for Low-Fat Varieties:** Low-fat options can help manage saturated fat intake.
- **Adopt portion control practices:** Stay mindful of the serving sizes, as even with healthy dairy options, overconsumption can potentially lead to weight gain.
- **Avoid Processed Dairy:** Stay away from highly processed products high in sodium and sugars. Refer to the "Go-To

Guide: Best Foods for the DiabeteBalance Diet" for approved cheeses.

- **Include Fermented Dairy:** Embrace plain yogurt and kefir for their probiotic benefits.
- **Watch for Added Sugars:** Check labels for added sugars, especially in flavored yogurts and processed cheeses.

Comprehensive Selection for the DiabeteBalance Diet:

Below is a list that aligns with the DiabeteBalance Diet, detailing serving size, Glycemic Index (GI), Glycemic Load (GL), and Net Carbohydrates. This vital information helps in informed decision-making for portion sizes and meal planning, organized alphabetically for ease of reference.

- 1% milk, (1 cup, 244g): GI of 27-45, GL of 5, Net carb= 12g

- 2% Greek Yogurt, (1 cup, 227g): GI of 11, GL of 4, Net carb= 10g

- 2% milk, (1 cup, 244g): GI of 27-45, GL of 5, Net carb= 12g

- Almond milk yogurt, (1 container (150g)): GI of <1, GL of <1, Net carb= 4g

- Almond milk, (1 cup, 240 ml): GI of <1, GL of <1, Net carb= 1g

- American Cheese, (1 oz, 28g): GI of 0, GL of 0, Net carb= 2g

- Appenzeller, (1 oz, 28g): GI of <1, GL of <1, Net carb= 0.1g

- Asiago Cheese, (1 oz, 28g): GI of 0, GL of 0, Net carb= 0g

- Asiago, (1 oz, 28g): GI of <1, GL of <1, Net carb= 0.9g

- Blue cheese, (1 oz, 28g): GI of <1, GL of <1, Net carb= 0.7g

- Brie Cheese, (1 oz, 28g): GI of 0, GL of 0, Net carb= 1g

- Burrata, (1 oz, 28g): GI of <1, GL of <1, Net carb= 1g

▦ Butter, (1 tbsp, 14g): GI of 0, GL of 0, Net carb= 0g

▦ Buttermilk, (1 cup, 245g): GI of 46, GL of 8, Net carb= 12g

▦ Camembert Cheese, (1 oz, 28g): GI of 0, GL of 0, Net carb= 0g

▦ Camembert, (1 oz, 28g): GI of <1, GL of <1, Net carb= 0.1g

▦ Cashew milk yogurt, (1 container (150g)): GI of <1, GL of <1, Net carb= 7g

▦ Cashew milk, (1 cup, 240 ml): GI of <1, GL of <1, Net carb= 2g

▦ Cheddar, (1 oz, 28g): GI of <1, GL of <1, Net carb= 0.4g

▦ Chèvre, (1 oz, 28g): GI of <1, GL of <1, Net carb= 0.2g

▦ Coconut milk yogurt, (1 container (150g)): GI of <1, GL of <1, Net carb= 5g

▦ Coconut milk, (1 cup, 240 ml): GI of <1, GL of <1, Net carb= 2g

▦ Colby Cheese, (1 oz, 28g): GI of 0, GL of 0, Net carb= 0g

▦ Colby Jack Cheese, (1 oz, 28g): GI of 0, GL of 0, Net carb= 1g

▦ Colby-Jack Cheese, (1 oz, 28g): GI of 0, GL of 0, Net carb= 0g

▦ Colby, (1 oz, 28g): GI of <1, GL of <1, Net carb= 0.7g

▦ Comté, (1 oz, 28g): GI of <1, GL of <1, Net carb= 0.4g

▦ Cottage Cheese, (1 cup, 226g): GI of 10, GL of 1, Net carb= 6g

▦ Cottage Cheese (Flavored), (1 cup, 226g): GI of 10, GL of 2, Net carb= 15g

▦ Cottage Cheese (Large Curd), (1 cup, 240g): GI of 10, GL of 2, Net carb= 10g

▦ Cottage Cheese (Low-fat), (1 cup, 226g): GI of 10, GL of 1, Net carb= 6g

▤ Cottage Cheese (Non-fat), (1 cup, 226g): GI of 10, GL of 1, Net carb= 10g

▤ Cottage Cheese (Small Curd), (1 cup, 240g): GI of 10, GL of 2, Net carb= 10g

▤ Cream Cheese, (1 oz, 28g): GI of 0, GL of 0, Net carb= 1g

▤ Cream Cheese (Flavored), (1 oz, 28g): GI of 0, GL of 0, Net carb= 2g

▤ Cream Cheese (Low-fat), (1 oz, 28g): GI of 0, GL of 0, Net carb= 1g

▤ Cream Cheese (Non-fat), (1 oz, 28g): GI of 0, GL of 0, Net carb= 2g

▤ Cream Cheese Spread, (1 tbsp, 14g): GI of 0, GL of 0, Net carb= 1g

▤ Creamer (Dairy-based), (1 tbsp, 15ml): GI of 47, GL of 1, Net carb= 5g

▤ Creamer (Non-dairy), (1 tbsp, 15ml): GI of 34, GL of 1, Net carb= 4g

▤ Edam Cheese, (1 oz, 28g): GI of 0, GL of 0, Net carb= 1g

▤ Emmental, (1 oz, 28g): GI of <1, GL of <1, Net carb= 0.4g

▤ Extra Firm Tofu, (1/2 cup, 126g): GI of 15, GL of 0, Net carb= 2g

▤ Farmer Cheese, (1 cup, 226g): GI of 10, GL of 2, Net carb= 10g

▤ Feta Cheese, (1 oz, 28g): GI of 0, GL of 0, Net carb= 1g

▤ Feta, (1 oz, 28g): GI of <1, GL of <1, Net carb= 1.2g

▤ Firm Tofu, (1/2 cup, 126g): GI of 15, GL of 0, Net carb= 2g

▤ Flax milk, (1 cup, 240 ml): GI of <1, GL of <1, Net carb= 1g

▤ Fontina, (1 oz, 28g): GI of <1, GL of <1, Net carb= 0.4g

▤ Ghee (Clarified Butter), (1 tbsp, 14g): GI of 0, GL of 0, Net carb= 0g

▤ Goat Cheese, (1 oz, 28g): GI of 0, GL of 0, Net carb= 1g

▤ Gorgonzola, (1 oz, 28g): GI of <1, GL of <1, Net carb= 0.3g

▤ Gouda Cheese, (1 oz, 28g): GI of 0, GL of 0, Net carb= 1g

▤ Greek Yogurt (Full-fat), (1 cup, 227g): GI of 11, GL of 5, Net carb= 10g

▤ Greek Yogurt (Low-fat), (1 cup, 227g): GI of 11, GL of 4, Net carb= 10g

▤ Greek Yogurt (Non-fat), (1 cup, 227g): GI of 11, GL of 3, Net carb= 10g

▤ Greek Yogurt (Plain), (1 cup, 227g): GI of 11, GL of 5, Net carb= 10g

▤ Gruyere Cheese, (1 oz, 28g): GI of 0, GL of 0, Net carb= 0g

▤ Half and Half, (1 tbsp, 15ml): GI of 0, GL of 0, Net carb= 0g

▤ Halloumi, (1 oz, 28g): GI of <1, GL of <1, Net carb= 1g

▤ Havarti Cheese, (1 oz, 28g): GI of 0, GL of 0, Net carb= 1g

▤ Hazelnut milk, (1 cup, 240 ml): GI of <1, GL of <1, Net carb= 2g

▤ Heavy Cream, (1 tbsp, 15ml): GI of 0, GL of 0, Net carb= 0g

▤ Hemp milk, (1 cup, 240 ml): GI of <1, GL of <1, Net carb= 2g

▤ Kefir, (1 cup, 240g): GI of 20, GL of 4, Net carb= 12g

▤ Labneh, (1 oz, 28g): GI of 0, GL of 0, Net carb= 2g

▤ Lactose-free milk, (1 cup, 244g): GI of 27-45, GL of 5, Net carb= 12g

▤ Limburger Cheese, (1 oz, 28g): GI of 0, GL of 0, Net carb= 0g

▤ Manchego, (1 oz, 28g): GI of <1, GL of <1, Net carb= 0g

▤ Mascarpone, (1 oz, 28g): GI of 0, GL of 0, Net carb= 1g

▤ Monterey Jack Cheese, (1 oz, 28g): GI of 0, GL of 0, Net carb= 1g

▤ Monterey Jack Cheese (with Jalapeño), (1 oz, 28g): GI of 0, GL of 0, Net carb= 1g

▤ Monterey Jack with Jalapeño, (1 oz, 28g): GI of <1, GL of <1, Net carb= 0.4g

▤ Monterey Jack, (1 oz, 28g): GI of <1, GL of <1, Net carb= 0.5g

▤ Mozzarella Cheese, (1 oz, 28g): GI of 0, GL of 0, Net carb= 1g

▤ Mozzarella, (1 oz, 28g): GI of <1, GL of <1, Net carb= 0.6g

▤ Muenster Cheese, (1 oz, 28g): GI of 0, GL of 0, Net carb= 0g

▤ Muenster, (1 oz, 28g): GI of <1, GL of <1, Net carb= 0.3g

▤ Neufchâtel Cheese, (1 oz, 28g): GI of 0, GL of 0, Net carb= 1g

▤ Non-fat Greek Yogurt, (1 cup, 227g): GI of 11, GL of 3, Net carb= 10g

▤ Organic milk, (1 cup, 244g): GI of 27-45, GL of 5, Net carb= 12g

▤ Panela Cheese, (1 oz, 28g): GI of 0, GL of 0, Net carb= 0g

▤ Parmesan, (1 oz, 28g): GI of <1, GL of <1, Net carb= 0.9g

▤ Pea milk, (1 cup (240 ml)): GI of 34, GL of 2, Net carb= 2g

▤ Pecorino Romano, (1 oz, 28g): GI of <1, GL of <1, Net carb= 0.5g

▤ Pepper Jack Cheese, (1 oz, 28g): GI of 0, GL of 0, Net carb= 1g

▤ Pepper Jack, (1 oz, 28g): GI of <1, GL of <1, Net carb= 0.5g

▤ Provolone Cheese, (1 oz, 28g): GI of 0, GL of 0, Net carb= 1g

▤ Provolone piccante, (1 oz, 28g): GI of <1, GL of <1, Net carb= 0.6g

▤ Provolone, (1 oz, 28g): GI of <1, GL of <1, Net carb= 0.6g

▤ Quark, (1 cup, 225g): GI of 0, GL of 0, Net carb= 9g

▤ Queso Blanco, (1 oz, 28g): GI of 0, GL of 0, Net carb= 0g

▤ Queso de Bola (Edam Cheese), (1 oz, 28g): GI of 0, GL of 0, Net carb= 0g

▤ Queso Fresco, (1 oz, 28g): GI of 0, GL of 0, Net carb= 0g

▤ Ricotta Cheese, (1 cup, 246g): GI of 0, GL of 0, Net carb= 7g

▤ Ricotta Cheese (Part-skim), (1 cup, 246g): GI of 0, GL of 0, Net carb= 7g

▤ Ricotta Cheese (Whole-milk), (1 cup, 246g): GI of 0, GL of 0, Net carb= 11g

▤ Ricotta Salata, (1 oz, 28g): GI of <1, GL of <1, Net carb= 1g

▤ Ricotta, (1/4 cup, 62g): GI of <1, GL of <1, Net carb= 3g

▤ Romano Cheese, (1 oz, 28g): GI of 0, GL of 0, Net carb= 0g

▤ Silken Tofu, (1/2 cup, 126g): GI of 15, GL of 0, Net carb= 1g

▤ Skim milk, (1 cup, 244g): GI of 27-45, GL of 4, Net carb= 12g

▤ Sour Cream, (1 cup, 230g): GI of 14, GL of 3, Net carb= 10g

▤ Sour Cream (Low-fat), (1 cup, 230g): GI of 14, GL of 3, Net carb= 10g

▤ Sour Cream (Non-fat), (1 cup, 230g): GI of 14, GL of 3, Net carb= 15g

▤ Soy Butter, (1 tbsp, 14g): GI of 0, GL of 0, Net carb= 0g

▤ Soy Cheese, (1 oz, 28g): GI of 14, GL of 0, Net carb= 0g

▤ Soy Cottage Cheese, (1 cup, 240g): GI of 15, GL of 3, Net carb= 5g

▤ Soy Cream Cheese, (1 oz, 28g): GI of 14, GL of 0, Net carb= 0g

▤ Soy Creamer, (1 tbsp, 15ml): GI of 34, GL of 1, Net carb= 2g

▤ Soy Milk (Plain), (1 cup, 240ml): GI of 34, GL of 4, Net carb= 4g

▦ Soy Milk (Unsweetened), (1 cup, 240ml): GI of 34, GL of 0, Net carb= 1g

▦ Soy Milk (Vanilla), (1 cup, 240ml): GI of 34, GL of 7, Net carb= 10g

▦ Soy milk, (1 cup, 240 ml): GI of 34, GL of 4, Net carb= 4g

▦ Soy Protein Powder, (1 scoop, 30g): GI of 25, GL of 6, Net carb= 2g

▦ Soy Ricotta Cheese, (1 cup, 246g): GI of 15, GL of 1, Net carb= 4g

▦ Soy Sour Cream, (1 tbsp, 14g): GI of 18, GL of 1, Net carb= 2g

▦ Soy Whipped Topping, (1 tbsp, 5g): GI of 0, GL of 0, Net carb= 0g

▦ Soy yogurt, (1 container (150g)): GI of 43, GL of 4, Net carb= 6g

▦ Soy Yogurt (Plain), (1 cup, 245g): GI of 32, GL of 9, Net carb= 15g

▦ Soy-based Coffee Creamer, (1 tbsp, 15ml): GI of 34, GL of 1, Net carb= 2g

▦ Soy-based Creamer (Flavored), (1 tbsp, 15ml): GI of 34, GL of 1, Net carb= 2g

▦ Soy-based Creamer (Non-dairy), (1 tbsp, 15ml): GI of 34, GL of 1, Net carb= 2g

▦ Soy-based Desserts, (1 serving, 100g): GI of 34, GL of 10, Net carb= 15g

▦ Soy-based Milkshake, (1 cup, 240ml): GI of 34, GL of 9, Net carb= 15g

▦ Soy-based Whipped Cream, (1 tbsp, 5g): GI of 0, GL of 0, Net carb= 0g

▦ Stilton Cheese, (1 oz, 28g): GI of 0, GL of 0, Net carb= 0g

▦ Stilton, (1 oz, 28g): GI of <1, GL of <1, Net carb= 0.4g

▦ Swiss Cheese, (1 oz, 28g): GI of 0, GL of 0, Net carb= 1g

▦ Swiss Cheese (Flavored), (1 oz, 28g): GI of 0, GL of 0, Net carb= 2g

▤ Swiss Cheese (Low-fat), (1 oz, 28g): GI of 0, GL of 0, Net carb= 1g

▤ Swiss Cheese (Non-fat), (1 oz, 28g): GI of 0, GL of 0, Net carb= 2g

▤ Swiss, (1 oz, 28g): GI of <1, GL of <1, Net carb= 1.5g

▤ Taleggio, (1 oz, 28g): GI of <1, GL of <1, Net carb= 0.1g

▤ Tempeh, (1 cup, 166g): GI of 35, GL of 5, Net carb= 10g

▤ Tofu, (1/2 cup, 126g): GI of 15, GL of 0, Net carb= 1g

▤ Whipped Butter, (1 tbsp, 14g): GI of 0, GL of 0, Net carb= 0g

▤ Whipped Cream, (1 cup, 240g): GI of 0, GL of 0, Net carb= 10g

▤ Whipped Topping, (1 cup, 76g): GI of 0, GL of 0, Net carb= 5g

▤ Whipped Topping (Light), (1 cup, 120g): GI of 0, GL of 0, Net carb= 10g

▤ Whole Milk Greek Yogurt, (1 cup, 227g): GI of 11, GL of 5, Net carb= 10g

▤ Whole milk, (1 cup (244g): GI of 27-45, GL of 5, Net carb= 12g

▤ Yogurt (Greek, Low-fat), (1 cup, 245g): GI of 11, GL of 5, Net carb= 10g

▤ Yogurt (Greek, Non-fat), (1 cup, 245g): GI of 11, GL of 4, Net carb= 10g

▤ Yogurt (Greek, Plain), (1 cup, 245g): GI of 11, GL of 5, Net carb= 10g

MEDIUM GLYCEMIC LOAD FOODS A-Z

In the DiabeteBalance Diet, we prioritize a strategic approach that empowers you to make informed dietary choices. While we emphasize foods with a low glycemic load as the adequate choice for optimally managing type 2 diabetes, we understand the need for variety and occasional indulgences.

Thus, we also provide comprehensive information on foods that fall within the medium glycemic load category. These are not the optimal option for regular consumption, but we believe in giving you a complete understanding of your options to help you navigate your food choices.

For each food item in this medium category, we present key details including typical serving size, Glycemic Index (GI), Glycemic Load (GL), and Net Carbohydrates. Armed with this information, you can make more conscious decisions even when you decide to consume these foods on occasion.

However, it's crucial to remember that portion control is vital when indulging in these foods. While they can be tolerated occasionally, we highly recommend reducing the standard serving size to ensure that your intake stays below 15 grams of net carbohydrates. This approach will help you maintain better blood sugar control while still allowing some flexibility in your diet.

▤ Caffè Mocha, (1 cup (240ml)): GI of 50, GL of 16, Net carb= 32g

▤ Caramel Latte, (1 cup (240ml)): GI of 50, GL of 12.5, Net carb= 25g

▤ Caramel Macchiato, (1 cup (240ml)): GI of 50, GL of 12.5, Net carb= 25g

▤ Chocolate Milk, (1 cup (240ml)): GI of 60, GL of 13.8, Net carb= 23g

▤ Coconut Milk, sweetened, (1 cup (240ml)): GI of 50, GL of 10.5, Net carb= 21g

▤ Hot Mocha, (1 cup (240ml)): GI of 50, GL of 15, Net carb= 30g

▤ Hot Peppermint Mocha, (1 cup (240ml)): GI of 50, GL of 15, Net carb= 30g

▤ Iced Chai Tea Latte, (1 cup (240ml)): GI of 50, GL of 12.5, Net carb= 25g

▤ Malt Drink, (1 cup (240ml)): GI of 50, GL of 17.5, Net carb= 35g

▤ Oat Milk, (1 cup (240ml)): GI of 69, GL of 16.6, Net carb= 24g

▤ Post-workout Recovery Drink, (1 cup (240ml)): GI of 50, GL of 12.5, Net carb= 25g

▤ Pre-workout Energy Drink, (1 cup (240ml)): GI of 65, GL of 19.5, Net carb= 30g

▤ Rice Milk, unsweetened, (1 cup (240ml)): GI of 75, GL of 11.3, Net carb= 15g

▤ Sarsaparilla, (1 cup (240ml)): GI of 50, GL of 12.5, Net carb= 25g

▤ Sports Drinks, (1 cup (240ml)): GI of 60, GL of 18, Net carb= 30g

▤ Tepache, (1 cup (240ml)): GI of 55, GL of 13.8, Net carb= 25g

▤ Thai Iced Tea, (1 cup (240ml)): GI of 50, GL of 12.5, Net carb= 25g

▤ Tiger Nut Milk, sweetened, (1 cup (240ml)): GI of 65, GL of 15.6, Net carb= 24g

▤ Tonic Water, (1 cup (240ml)): GI of 50, GL of 12.5, Net carb= 25g

▤ Yogurt Smoothie, (1 cup (240ml)): GI of 50, GL of 15, Net carb= 30g

DIPS AND DRESSINGS

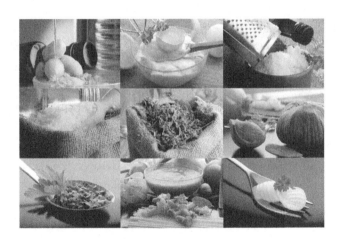

Dips and dressings are more than mere condiments; they can elevate the flavors of dishes while contributing to a balanced diet. When following the DiabeteBalance Diet, attention must be paid to selecting those that comply with principles such as low glycemic load (GL), the Mediterranean Diet, the 2020-2025 Dietary Guidelines for Americans, and the twin cycle hypothesis.

Benefits of Suitable Dips and Dressings:

- **Flavor Enhancer:** By augmenting the taste of meals, dips and dressings can make nutrient-rich food more appealing.
- **Nutrient Intake:** Dips and dressings made with healthy fats (e.g., avocados, olive oil) or nutrient-dense foods (e.g., yogurt) provide additional vitamins, minerals, and beneficial fats.

Potential Drawbacks:

- **High Sodium Content:** Some commercially prepared products may contain excessive sodium, a risk factor for high blood pressure.
- **High Fat Content:** Creamy or cheese-based options might be high in saturated fat, potentially affecting heart health.
- **High Glycemic Impact:** Products with added sugars or high-GI foods can lead to elevated blood glucose levels.

Guidelines for Incorporating Dips and Dressings into the Diabete-Balance Diet:

- **Check the Labels:** Look for products low in sodium, sugar, and unhealthy fats by reading the nutrition facts and ingredient lists.
- **Portion Control:** Adhere to recommended serving sizes, as even healthy options can add substantial calories and fats if overconsumed.
- **Make Your Own:** Creating homemade dips and dressings ensures control over the ingredients, often resulting in more nutritious and less processed choices.

Comprehensive Selection for the DiabeteBalance Diet:

Below is an alphabetical list of foods that comply with the DiabeteBalance Diet. Details on serving size, Glycemic Index (GI), Glycemic

Load (GL), and Net Carbohydrates are included, empowering you with the knowledge needed for smart decision-making on portion sizes and meal planning.

▤ Artichoke Dip, (1 tbsp, 15 ml): GI of 40-45, GL of 1, Net carb= 2.2g

▤ Asian Sesame Dressing, (2 tbsp, 30 mL): GI of 30-45, GL of 1.4, Net carb= 3g

▤ Avocado Lime Dressing, (2 tbsp, 30 mL): GI of 30-45, GL of 0.4, Net carb= 1g

▤ Avocado Ranch Dressing, (2 tbsp, 30 mL): GI of 45-50, GL of 1, Net carb= 2g

▤ Baba Ghanoush, (2 tbsp, 30g): GI of 40-50, GL of 1, Net carb= 2g

▤ Bacon Ranch Dip, (1 tbsp, 15 ml): GI of 25-30, GL of 0.4, Net carb= 1g

▤ Balsamic Vinaigrette, (2 tbsp, 30 mL): GI of 50-55, GL of 1.1, Net carb= 2g

▤ Black Bean Dip, (2 tbsp, 30g): GI of 30-35, GL of 1.2, Net carb= 3g

▤ Blue Cheese Dressing, (1 tbsp, 15 mL): GI of 45-50, GL of 0.5, Net carb= 1g

▤ Buffalo Cauliflower Dip, (1 tbsp, 15 ml): GI of 35-40, GL of 0.8, Net carb= 2g

▤ Buffalo Chicken Dip, (2 tbsp, 30g): GI of 30-35, GL of 0.7, Net carb= 2g

▤ Caesar Dressing, (2 tbsp, 30 mL): GI of 45-50, GL of 1, Net carb= 1g

▤ Champagne Vinaigrette, (2 tbsp, 30 mL): GI of 40-50, GL of 1, Net carb= 2g

▤ Cheese Dip, (1 tbsp, 15 ml): GI of 30-35, GL of 0.3, Net carb= 1g

▤ Chimichurri Sauce, (2 tbsp, 30 mL): GI of 30-45, GL of 0.5, Net carb= 1g

▤ Chipotle Lime Dressing, (2 tbsp, 30 mL): GI of 30-45, GL of 0.5, Net carb= 1g

▤ Cilantro Lime Dip, (1 tbsp, 15 ml): GI of 25-30, GL of 0.3, Net carb= 1g

▤ Clam Dip, (1 tbsp, 15 ml): GI of 25-30, GL of 0.3, Net carb= 1g

▤ Corn Dip, (1 tbsp, 15 ml): GI of 55-60, GL of 2.5, Net carb= 4.2g

▤ Creamy Garlic Dressing, (2 tbsp, 30 mL): GI of 30-45, GL of 0.5, Net carb= 1g

▤ Creamy Italian Dressing, (2 tbsp, 30 mL): GI of 30-45, GL of 0.5, Net carb= 1g

▤ Creamy Ranch Dressing, (2 tbsp, 30 mL): GI of 30-45, GL of 0.5, Net carb= 1g

▤ Cucumber Dill Dressing, (2 tbsp, 30 mL): GI of 30-45, GL of 0.5, Net carb= 1g

▤ Cucumber Dip, (1 tbsp, 15 ml): GI of 20-25, GL of 0.2, Net carb= 0.8g

▤ Deviled Egg Dip, (1 tbsp, 15 ml): GI of 20-25, GL of 0.1, Net carb= 0.5g

▤ Edamame Dip, (1 tbsp, 15 ml): GI of 20-25, GL of 0.3, Net carb= 1.2g

▤ Fava Bean Dip, (1 tbsp, 15 ml): GI of 30-40, GL of 0.8, Net carb= 2g

▤ Feta Dip, (1 tbsp, 15 ml): GI of 20-25, GL of 0.1, Net carb= 0.5g

▤ Ginger Soy Dip, (1 tbsp, 15 ml): GI of 25-30, GL of 0.3, Net carb= 1g

▤ Gochujang Dressing, (1 tbsp, 15 mL): GI of 30-45, GL of 0.5, Net carb= 1g

▤ Gouda Dip, (1 tbsp, 15 ml): GI of 20-25, GL of 0.1, Net carb= 0.5g

▤ Greek Yogurt Dip, (1 tbsp, 15 ml): GI of 25-30, GL of 0.3, Net carb= 1.2g

▤ Green Goddess Dip, (1 tbsp, 15 ml): GI of 20-25, GL of 0.3, Net carb= 1g

▤ Hoisin Dip, (1 tbsp, 15 ml): GI of 40-50, GL of 1.1, Net carb= 2.2g

▤ Horseradish Dip, (1 tbsp, 15 ml): GI of 25-30, GL of 0.3, Net carb= 1g

▤ Hot Crab Dip, (1 tbsp, 15 ml): GI of 20-25, GL of 0.1, Net carb= 0.7g

▤ Hummus, (2 tbsp, 30g): GI of 30-35, GL of 1.4, Net carb= 4g

▤ Italian Dressing, (1 tbsp, 15 mL): GI of 30-50, GL of 0.5, Net carb= 1g

▤ Jalapeño Popper Dip, (2 tbsp, 30g): GI of 30-35, GL of 0.7, Net carb= 2g

▤ Lemon Vinaigrette, (2 tbsp, 30 mL): GI of 30-45, GL of 0.4, Net carb= 1g

▤ Mango Chutney Dip, (1 tbsp, 15 ml): GI of 40-50, GL of 1.5, Net carb= 3g

▤ Mango Salsa, (1 tbsp, 15 ml): GI of 40-50, GL of 1.5, Net carb= 3g

▤ Mexican Street Corn Dip, (1 tbsp, 15 ml): GI of 55-60, GL of 2.1, Net carb= 4g

▤ Mustard Dip, (1 tbsp, 15 ml): GI of 20-25, GL of 0.1, Net carb= 0.8g

▤ Nacho Dip, (1 tbsp, 15 ml): GI of 30-35, GL of 0.5, Net carb= 1.2g

▤ Olive Tapenade, (1 tbsp, 15 ml): GI of 15-20, GL of 0.2, Net carb= 0.8g

▤ Onion Dip, (1 tbsp, 15 ml): GI of 25-30, GL of 0.4, Net carb= 1g

▤ Peanut Butter Dip, (1 tbsp, 15 ml): GI of 40-55, GL of 1.2, Net carb= 2.2g

▤ Pesto Dip, (1 tbsp, 15 ml): GI of 20-30, GL of 0.3, Net carb= 1g

▤ Pico de Gallo, (2 tbsp, 30g): GI of 20-25, GL of 0.5, Net carb= 2g

▤ Pineapple Salsa, (1 tbsp, 15 ml): GI of 40-55, GL of 1.5, Net carb= 3g

▤ Roasted Eggplant Dip, (1 tbsp, 15 ml): GI of 30-45, GL of 0.8, Net carb= 1.5g

▤ Roasted Garlic Dip, (1 tbsp, 15 ml): GI of 30-40, GL of 0.8, Net carb= 1.5g

▤ Roasted Red Pepper Dip, (1 tbsp, 15 ml): GI of 35-40, GL of 0.9, Net carb= 2g

▤ Roasted Tomato Dip, (1 tbsp, 15 ml): GI of 30-35, GL of 0.5, Net carb= 1.2g

▤ Roquefort Cheese Dressing, (2 tbsp, 30 mL): GI of 40-50, GL of 0.5, Net carb= 2g

▤ Salmon Dip, (1 tbsp, 15 ml): GI of 20-25, GL of 0.1, Net carb= 0.5g

▤ Shrimp Dip, (1 tbsp, 15 ml): GI of 20-25, GL of 0.1, Net carb= 0.5g

▤ Smoked Gouda Dip, (1 tbsp, 15 ml): GI of 20-25, GL of 0.1, Net carb= 0.5g

▤ Smoked Salmon Dip, (1 tbsp, 15 ml): GI of 20-25, GL of 0.1, Net carb= 0.5g

▤ Smoky Red Pepper Dip, (1 tbsp, 15 ml): GI of 35-40, GL of 0.9, Net carb= 2g

▤ Southwestern Dip, (1 tbsp, 15 ml): GI of 30-40, GL of 0.8, Net carb= 1.5g

▤ Spicy Pimiento Cheese Dip, (1 tbsp, 15 ml): GI of 35-50, GL of 0.9, Net carb= 1.5g

▤ Sweet Potato Dip, (1 tbsp, 15 ml): GI of 50-55, GL of 1.6, Net carb= 3g

▤ Tapenade, (1 tbsp, 15 ml): GI of 15-20, GL of 0.1, Net carb= 0.8g

▤ Teriyaki Dip, (1 tbsp, 15 ml): GI of 40-55, GL of 1.2, Net carb= 2.2g

▤ Tex-Mex Dip, (1 tbsp, 15 ml): GI of 30-45, GL of 0.8, Net carb= 1.5g

▤ Thai Peanut Dip, (1 tbsp, 15 ml): GI of 40-55, GL of 0.6, Net carb= 2.2g

▤ Tomato Basil Dip, (1 tbsp, 15 ml): GI of 25-30, GL of 0.3, Net carb= 1g

▤ Tuna Dip, (1 tbsp, 15 ml): GI of 20-25, GL of 0.1, Net carb= 0.5g

▤ Wasabi Dip, (1 tbsp, 15 ml): GI of 20-25, GL of 0.1, Net carb= 0.5g

▤ Whipped Feta Dip, (1 tbsp, 15 ml): GI of 20-25, GL of 0.1, Net carb= 0.5g

▤ Whipped Goat Cheese Dip, (1 tbsp, 15 ml): GI of 20-25, GL of 0.1, Net carb= 0.5g

▤ White Queso Dip, (1 tbsp, 15 ml): GI of 30-35, GL of 0.4, Net carb= 1g

▤ Zucchini Dip, (1 tbsp, 15 ml): GI of 20-25, GL of 0.2, Net carb= 1g

GRAINS, CEREALS AND PASTA

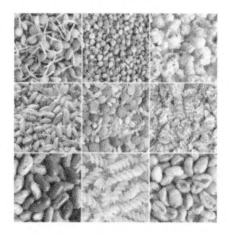

Grains and cereals are staples in many diets worldwide, and their role within the DiabeteBalance Diet must be carefully considered. Understanding their glycemic load (GL), nutritional content, and alignment with the DiabeteBalance Diet principles is vital for supporting diabetes management and overall well-being.

Benefits of Grains and Cereals:

- **Nutrient-Dense:** Whole grains and cereals are packed with essential nutrients such as dietary fiber, B vitamins, iron, magnesium, and selenium.
- **Source of Fiber:** Whole grains offer valuable dietary fiber, which helps regulate sugar absorption, thus moderating glucose and insulin levels.

Potential Drawbacks:

- **Refined Grains:** Stripped of their nutrient-rich outer layers, refined grains like white rice and bread can cause rapid spikes in blood sugar.
- **High in Carbohydrates:** The carbohydrate-rich nature of grains and cereals may affect blood sugar levels if consumed without proper portion control.

Guidelines for Incorporating Grains and Cereals into the Diabete-Balance Diet:

- **Opt for Whole Grains:** Emphasize whole grains such as brown rice, oatmeal, quinoa, and whole-grain bread or pasta, as they have a lower GL compared to refined alternatives.
- **Monitor Portion Sizes:** Due to their carbohydrate content, mindful portioning of grains and cereals can assist in blood sugar management and weight control.
- **Read Labels Diligently:** Carefully review labels when shopping for grain products, focusing on those listing whole grains as primary ingredients and avoiding added sugars.

Comprehensive Selection for the DiabeteBalance Diet:

Below is an alphabetical listing of foods that align with the Diabete-Balance Diet. Detailed information on serving size, Glycemic Index

(GI), Glycemic Load (GL), and Net Carbohydrates is provided, arming you with the insights needed to make educated choices for portion sizes and meal planning.

LOW GLYCEMIC LOAD FOODS A-Z

▤ Amaranth, (½ cup cooked, 123g): GI of 35, GL of 3.5, Net carb= 10g

▤ Barley, (½ cup cooked, 89g): GI of 28, GL of 4.5, Net carb= 16g

▤ Barley Hulled, (½ cup cooked, 89g): GI of 25-30, GL of 5.5, Net carb= 20g

▤ Bhutanese Red Rice, (½ cup cooked, 92g): GI of 45, GL of 9.4, Net carb= 19.2g

▤ Black Rice, (½ cup cooked, 93g): GI of 44, GL of 9.7, Net carb= 16g

▤ Brown Rice Porridge, (½ cup cooked, 98g): GI of 55-70, GL of 7.5, Net carb= 16g

▤ Buckwheat, (½ cup cooked, 84g): GI of 45-55, GL of 7.5, Net carb= 16.5g

▤ Buckwheat Groats, (½ cup cooked, 84g): GI of 45, GL of 6.5, Net carb= 14.5g

▤ Buckwheat Noodles, (½ cup cooked, 57g): GI of 45, GL of 9.5, Net carb= 21g

▤ Buckwheat Porridge, (½ cup cooked, 84g): GI of 50-65, GL of 7, Net carb= 11.5g

▤ Buckwheat Spaghetti, (½ cup cooked, 70g): GI of 45, GL of 9.5, Net carb= 21g

▤ Bulgur, (½ cup cooked, 91g): GI of 46, GL of 6, Net carb= 13g

▤ Canned Hominy, (½ cup, 82g): GI of 40-45, GL of 6, Net carb= 12g

▤ Corn Bran Crude, (½ cup, 30g): GI of 40-45, GL of 4.5, Net carb= 9.5g

▤ Eggplant Lasagna, (½ cup, 1200g): GI of 50, GL of 5, Net carb= 10g

▤ Four Cheese Lasagna, (½ cup, 120g): GI of 50, GL of 4, Net carb= 10g

▤ Freekeh, (½ cup cooked, 81g): GI of 43, GL of 6, Net carb= 14g

▤ Grits, (½ cup cooked, 121g): GI of 60-80, GL of 7.5, Net carb= 14g

▤ Hominy Canned Yellow, (½ cup, 82g): GI of 40-45, GL of 6, Net carb= 12g

▤ Hulled Barley, (½ cup cooked, 78g): GI of 28, GL of 4.5, Net carb= 16g

▤ Japanese Somen, (½ cup, 73g): GI of 45-50, GL of 9.5, Net carb= 19g

▤ Kamut Pasta, (½ cup cooked, 70g): GI of 45-50, GL of 10, Net carb= 21g

▤ Mexican Lasagna, (½ cup, 120g): GI of 50, GL of 7.5, Net carb= 17.5g

▤ Millet Porridge, (½ cup cooked, 100g): GI of 50-70, GL of 7, Net carb= 12g

▤ Oat Bran, (½ cup, 110g): GI of 55-60, GL of 5.5, Net carb= 12g

▤ Oatmeal, (½ cup cooked, 117g): GI of 55-65, GL of 8.5, Net carb= 13.5g

▤ Oatmeal, (½ cup, 117g): GI of 55-60, GL of 7, Net carb= 15g

▤ Pesto Lasagna, (½ cup, 120g): GI of 50, GL of 5, Net carb= 15g

▤ Polenta, (½ cup cooked, 64g): GI of 70-85, GL of 9, Net carb= 12g

▤ Popcorn, (3 cups popped, 24g): GI of 55-65, GL of 7, Net carb= 15g

Quinoa, (½ cup cooked, 185g): GI of 53, GL of 5, Net carb= 17g

Quinoa Porridge, (½ cup cooked, 93g): GI of 50-65, GL of 6.5, Net carb= 11.5g

Rice Bran, (½ cup, 58g): GI of 20-25, GL of 3, Net carb= 9g

Rye, (1 slice of bread, 32g): GI of 57-62, GL of 10, Net carb= 14g

Rye Grain, (½ cup cooked, 87g): GI of 45-50, GL of 7, Net carb= 15g

Seafood Lasagna, (½ cup, 240g): GI of 50, GL of 5, Net carb= 12.5g

Semolina Porridge, (½ cup cooked, 83g): GI of 50-65, GL of 6.5, Net carb= 11g

Shirataki Spaghetti, (1 cup, 160g): GI of 0, GL of 0, Net carb= 0g

Soba, (½ cup cooked, 57g): GI of 45, GL of 9.5, Net carb= 21g

Sorghum, (½ cup cooked, 96g): GI of 65, GL of 9.5, Net carb= 14.5g

Spelt Pasta, (½ cup cooked, 70g): GI of 44-49, GL of 9.5, Net carb= 20.5g

Spinach Lasagna, (½ cup, 120g): GI of 50, GL of 6, Net carb= 15g

Steel-Cut Oats, (½ cup cooked, 120g): GI of 55, GL of 7.5, Net carb= 13.5g

Teff, (½ cup, 126g): GI of 45-50, GL of 8.5, Net carb= 21g

Teff Porridge, (½ cup cooked, 120g): GI of 60-75, GL of 9, Net carb= 14.5g

Traditional Lasagna, (½ cup, 120g): GI of 50, GL of 7, Net carb= 18g

Triticale, (½ cup cooked, 182g): GI of 45-50, GL of 9.5, Net carb= 20g

▤ Vegetarian Lasagna, (½ cup, 120g): GI of 50, GL of 5, Net carb= 12.5g

▤ Vermicelli Made from Soybeans, (½ cup cooked, 150g): GI of 20-25, GL of 2.5, Net carb= 6g

▤ Wheat Bran Crude, (1 cup, 58g): GI of 40-45, GL of 7, Net carb= 20g

▤ Wheat Germ Crude, (½ cup, 58g): GI of 40-45, GL of 7.5, Net carb= 19.5g

▤ Wheat Sprouted, (½ cup, 55g): GI of 45-50, GL of 8.5, Net carb= 15.5g

▤ Wild Barley, (½ cup cooked, 87g): GI of 28-35, GL of 5, Net carb= 18g

▤ Wild Rice, (½ cup cooked, 82g): GI of 45-55, GL of 8, Net carb= 16g

MEDIUM GLYCEMIC LOAD FOODS A-Z

In the DiabeteBalance Diet, we prioritize a strategic approach that empowers you to make informed dietary choices. While we emphasize foods with a low glycemic load as the adequate choice for optimally managing type 2 diabetes, we understand the need for variety and occasional indulgences.

Thus, we also provide comprehensive information on foods that fall within the medium glycemic load category. These are not the optimal option for regular consumption, but we believe in giving you a complete understanding of your options to help you navigate your food choices.

For each food item in this medium category, we present key details including typical serving size, Glycemic Index (GI), Glycemic Load

(GL), and Net Carbohydrates. Armed with this information, you can make more conscious decisions even when you decide to consume these foods on occasion.

However, it's crucial to remember that portion control is vital when indulging in these foods. While they can be tolerated occasionally, we highly recommend reducing the standard serving size to ensure that your intake stays below 15 grams of net carbohydrates. This approach will help you maintain better blood sugar control while still allowing some flexibility in your diet.

▤ Angel Hair Spaghetti, (½ cup cooked, 70g): GI of 45, GL of 11, Net carb= 25g

▤ Arborio Rice, (½ cup cooked, 100g): GI of 70, GL of 17.5, Net carb= 25g

▤ Basmati Rice, (½ cup cooked, 80g): GI of 58, GL of 12, Net carb= 19g

▤ Brown Basmati Rice, (½ cup cooked, 97g): GI of 55, GL of 10.5, Net carb= 19g

▤ Brown Jasmine Rice, (½ cup cooked, 97g): GI of 55, GL of 11.5, Net carb= 17g

▤ Brown Rice, (½ cup cooked, 98g): GI of 55, GL of 10.5, Net carb= 19g

▤ Brown Rice Noodles, (½ cup cooked, 90g): GI of 65, GL of 13, Net carb= 20g

▤ Bucatini, (½ cup cooked, 70g): GI of 55, GL of 12.2, Net carb= 25g

▤ Capellini, (½ cup cooked, 70g): GI of 55, GL of 13.75, Net carb= 25g

▤ Carnaroli Rice, (½ cup cooked, 100g): GI of 70, GL of 17.5, Net carb= 25g

▤ Carrot Spaghetti, (½ cup cooked, 70g): GI of 45, GL of 11, Net carb= 24.5g

▤ Chow Mein Noodles, (½ cup cooked, 70g): GI of 45, GL of 11, Net carb= 23g

▤ Congee, (½ cup cooked, 125g): GI of 75, GL of 15, Net carb= 22.5g

▤ Corn Grain White, (½ cup boiled, 164g): GI of 55-60, GL of 13.5, Net carb= 22.5g

▤ Corn Grain Yellow, (1 cup boiled, 164g): GI of 55-60, GL of 13.5, Net carb= 22.5g

▤ Cornmeal, (¼ cup dry, 30g): GI of 69, GL of 15, Net carb= 20g

▤ Couscous, (½ cup cooked, 79g): GI of 65, GL of 11, Net carb= 18g

▤ Egg Noodles, (½ cup cooked, 70g): GI of 40, GL of 10, Net carb= 25g

▤ Farro, (½ cup cooked, 84g): GI of 40, GL of 9, Net carb= 22g

▤ Mushroom Lasagna, (½ cup, 120g): GI of 50, GL of 6.5, Net carb= 16.5g

▤ Rice Noodles, (½ cup cooked, 85g): GI of 55, GL of 11, Net carb= 20g

FISH, SEAFOOD, AND FISH PRODUCTS

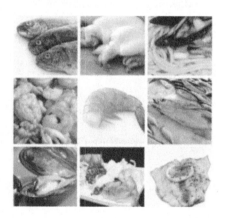

Fish and seafood are pivotal elements in numerous diets and provide unique advantages for those adhering to the DiabeteBalance Diet. While fish are typically low in carbs, the cooking method can affect their nutritional profile. It's vital to evaluate their glycemic load (GL), nutritional values, and suitability within the diet. Grasping the benefits and possible concerns related to fish, seafood, and their by-products enables individuals to make enlightened decisions that bolster diabetes control and holistic well-being.

Benefits of Fish and Seafood:

- **Rich in Omega-3:** Oily fish, like anchovies, herring, salmon, mackerel, and sardines, serve as prime sources of omega-3 fatty acids, which offer significant benefits for heart health.
- **High-Quality Protein:** Fish and seafood supply high-quality protein that helps maintain muscle mass and satiety.
- **Low Glycemic Load:** Fish and seafood typically have a low GL, meaning a minimal impact on blood sugar levels.
- **Key Nutrients:** These foods offer essential nutrients like omega-3, vitamin D, and vitamin E, aiding in stable blood sugar and insulin regulation.

Potential Drawbacks:

- **Mercury Levels:** Some fish, especially larger predatory varieties like swordfish and tuna, may contain high mercury levels.
- **Cooking Methods:** Methods such as deep frying can add unhealthy fats and increase the GL, while breading or flouring may also elevate glycemic load.
- **Fish By-Products:** Highly processed products like fish nuggets or sticks often contain unhealthy additives and excessive sodium.

Guidelines for Incorporating Fish and Seafood into the Diabete-Balance Diet:

- **Opt for Low-Mercury Fish:** Favor low-mercury options like salmon, sardines, and trout.
- **Healthy Cooking Methods:** Choose healthier cooking techniques such as grilling, baking, broiling, or steaming, avoiding frying or methods involving substantial added fats.

Comprehensive Selection for the DiabeteBalance Diet:

Below is an alphabetical listing of foods that align with the Diabete-Balance Diet. The provided details on serving size, Glycemic Index (GI), Glycemic Load (GL), and Net Carbohydrates equip you with the insights necessary for informed decision-making on portion sizes and meal planning.

▤ Albacore Tuna, (3 oz (85g)): GI of 0, GL of 0, Net carb= 0g

▤ Amberjack, (3 oz (85g)): GI of 0, GL of 0, Net carb= 0g

▤ Anchovies, (3 oz (85g)): GI of 0, GL of 0, Net carb= 0g

▤ Barramundi, (3 oz (85g)): GI of 0, GL of 0, Net carb= 0g

▤ Black Drum, (3 oz (85g)): GI of 0, GL of 0, Net carb= 0g

▤ Black Sea Bass, (3 oz (85g)): GI of 0, GL of 0, Net carb= 0g

▤ Blackfin Tuna, (3 oz (85g)): GI of 0, GL of 0, Net carb= 0g

▤ Bluefin Tuna, (3 oz (85g)): GI of 0, GL of 0, Net carb= 0g

▤ Bluefish, (3 oz (85g)): GI of 0, GL of 0, Net carb= 0g

▤ Cajun Spiced Salmon Salad, low-carb dressing, (7oz (200g)): GI of 45, GL of 4, Net carb= 9g

▤ Canned Mackerel (in water), (3 oz (85g)): GI of 0, GL of 0, Net carb= 0g

▤ Canned Salmon (in water), (3 oz (85g)): GI of 0, GL of 0, Net carb= 0g

▤ Canned Sardines (in water), (3 oz (85g)): GI of 0, GL of 0, Net carb= 0g

▤ Canned Trout (in water), (3 oz (85g)): GI of 0, GL of 0, Net carb= 0g

▤ Canned Tuna (in water), (3 oz (85g)): GI of 0, GL of 0, Net carb= 1g

▤ Catfish, (3 oz (85g)): GI of 0, GL of 0, Net carb= 0g

▤ Caviar, (1 tbsp (16g)): GI of 0, GL of 0, Net carb= 0g

▤ Ceviche Salad, (7oz (200g)): GI of 40, GL of 2, Net carb= 6g

▤ Clams, (3 oz (85g)): GI of 0, GL of 0, Net carb= 2g

▤ Cobia, (3 oz (85g)): GI of 0, GL of 0, Net carb= 0g

▤ Cod, (3 oz (85g)): GI of 0, GL of 0, Net carb= 0g

▤ Crab, (3 oz (85g)): GI of 0, GL of 0, Net carb= 0g

▤ Crab and Avocado Salad, low-carb dressing, (7oz (200g)): GI of 35, GL of 2, Net carb= 5g

▤ Crab and Mango Salad, low-carb dressing, (7oz (200g)): GI of 35, GL of 2, Net carb= 6g

▤ Crab and Watermelon Salad, low-carb dressing, (7oz (200g)): GI of 40, GL of 2, Net carb= 6g

▤ Crab Louie Salad, low-carb dressing, (8oz (250g)): GI of 35, GL of 2, Net carb= 7g

▤ Crab Quinoa Salad, low-carb dressing, (7oz (200g)): GI of 35, GL of 2, Net carb= 6g

▤ Crayfish, (3 oz (85g)): GI of 0, GL of 0, Net carb= 0g

▤ Croaker, (3 oz (85g)): GI of 0, GL of 0, Net carb= 0g

▤ Drum, (3 oz (85g)): GI of 0, GL of 0, Net carb= 0g

▤ Fish and Chips, (1 serving (350g)): GI of 55, GL of 50, Net carb= 90g

▤ Fish and Vegetable Skewers, (1 skewer (100g)): GI of 55, GL of 8, Net carb= 15g

▤ Fish Ball, (1 ball (25g)): GI of 55, GL of 2, Net carb= 3g

▤ Fish Burger, (1 patty (85g)): GI of 55, GL of 12, Net carb= 22g

▤ Fish Fillet, (1 fillet (85g)): GI of 55, GL of 12, Net carb= 22g

▤ Fish Patty Sandwich, (1 sandwich (200g)): GI of 55, GL of 17, Net carb= 30g

▤ Fish Sandwich, (1 sandwich (200g)): GI of 55, GL of 22, Net carb= 40g

▤ Fish Taco, (1 taco (150g)): GI of 55, GL of 14, Net carb= 26g

▤ Fish Tacos, (1 taco (150g)): GI of 55, GL of 14, Net carb= 26g

▤ Fish Wrap, (1 wrap (200g)): GI of 55, GL of 22, Net carb= 40g

▤ Flounder, (3 oz (85g)): GI of 0, GL of 0, Net carb= 0g

▤ Greek Salmon Salad, low-carb dressing, (7oz (200g)): GI of 40, GL of 3, Net carb= 8g

▤ Grilled Shrimp and Quinoa Salad, (7oz (200g)): GI of 40, GL of 3, Net carb= 8g

▤ Grouper, (3 oz (85g)): GI of 0, GL of 0, Net carb= 0g

▤ Haddock, (3 oz (85g)): GI of 0, GL of 0, Net carb= 0g

▤ Halibut, (3 oz (85g)): GI of 0, GL of 0, Net carb= 0g

▤ Herring, (3 oz (85g)): GI of 0, GL of 0, Net carb= 0g

▤ King Mackerel, (3 oz (85g)): GI of 0, GL of 0, Net carb= 0g

▤ Lake Trout, (3 oz (85g)): GI of 0, GL of 0, Net carb= 0g

▤ Lingcod, (3 oz (85g)): GI of 0, GL of 0, Net carb= 0g

▤ Lobster, (3 oz (85g)): GI of 0, GL of 0, Net carb= 0g

▤ Lobster Cobb Salad, (8oz (250g)): GI of 40, GL of 3, Net carb= 8g

▤ Lobster Mango Salad, (7oz (200g)): GI of 35, GL of 2, Net carb= 7g

▤ Mackerel, (3 oz (85g)): GI of 0, GL of 0, Net carb= 0g

▤ Marlin, (3 oz (85g)): GI of 0, GL of 0, Net carb= 0g

▦ Mediterranean Octopus Salad, low-carb dressing, (7oz (200g)): GI of 40, GL of 2, Net carb= 6g

▦ Monkfish, (3 oz (85g)): GI of 0, GL of 0, Net carb= 0g

▦ Mussels, (3 oz (85g)): GI of 0, GL of 0, Net carb= 3g

▦ Octopus, (3 oz (85g)): GI of 0, GL of 0, Net carb= 0g

▦ Oysters, (3 oz (85g)): GI of 0, GL of 0, Net carb= 3g

▦ Parrotfish, (3 oz (85g)): GI of 0, GL of 0, Net carb= 0g

▦ Pink Snapper, (3 oz (85g)): GI of 0, GL of 0, Net carb= 0g

▦ Pollock, (3 oz (85g)): GI of 0, GL of 0, Net carb= 0g

▦ Pompano, (3 oz (85g)): GI of 0, GL of 0, Net carb= 0g

▦ Rainbow Trout, (3 oz (85g)): GI of 0, GL of 0, Net carb= 0g

▦ Red Drum, (3 oz (85g)): GI of 0, GL of 0, Net carb= 0g

▦ Red Snapper, (3 oz (85g)): GI of 0, GL of 0, Net carb= 0g

▦ Redfish, (3 oz (85g)): GI of 0, GL of 0, Net carb= 0g

▦ Rockfish, (3 oz (85g)): GI of 0, GL of 0, Net carb= 0g

▦ Sablefish, (3 oz (85g)): GI of 0, GL of 0, Net carb= 0g

▦ Salmon, (3 oz (85g)): GI of 0, GL of 0, Net carb= 0g

▦ Salmon Caesar Salad, low-carb dressing, (7oz (200g)): GI of 45, GL of 4, Net carb= 8g

▦ Salmon Spinach Salad, low-carb dressing, (7oz (200g)): GI of 40, GL of 3, Net carb= 7g

▦ Sardines, (3 oz (85g)): GI of 0, GL of 0, Net carb= 0g

▦ Scallop Salad, low-carb dressing, (7oz (200g)): GI of 40, GL of 2, Net carb= 5g

▦ Scallops, (3 oz (85g)): GI of 0, GL of 0, Net carb= 2g

▤ Seared Ahi Tuna Salad, (7oz (200g)): GI of 40, GL of 3, Net carb= 7g

▤ Seared Scallop and Grapefruit Salad, low-carb dressing, (7oz (200g)): GI of 35, GL of 2, Net carb= 5g

▤ Seared Scallops and Asparagus Salad, low-carb dressing, (7oz (200g)): GI of 35, GL of 2, Net carb= 5g

▤ Seared Swordfish Salad, (7oz (200g)): GI of 40, GL of 3, Net carb= 7g

▤ Sheepshead, (3 oz (85g)): GI of 0, GL of 0, Net carb= 0g

▤ Shrimp, (3 oz (85g)): GI of 0, GL of 0, Net carb= 0g

▤ Shrimp Avocado Salad, low-carb dressing, (7oz (200g)): GI of 35, GL of 2, Net carb= 6g

▤ Shrimp Cobb Salad, (7oz (200g)): GI of 40, GL of 3, Net carb= 8g

▤ Skate, (3 oz (85g)): GI of 0, GL of 0, Net carb= 0g

▤ Spicy Tuna Salad, low-carb dressing, (7oz (200g)): GI of 45, GL of 3, Net carb= 7g

▤ Squid, (3 oz (85g)): GI of 0, GL of 0, Net carb= 0g

▤ Striped Bass, (3 oz (85g)): GI of 0, GL of 0, Net carb= 0g

▤ Striped Marlin, (3 oz (85g)): GI of 0, GL of 0, Net carb= 0g

▤ Surimi, (3 oz (85g)): GI of 25, GL of 1, Net carb= 5g

▤ Swordfish, (3 oz (85g)): GI of 0, GL of 0, Net carb= 0g

▤ Tautog, (3 oz (85g)): GI of 0, GL of 0, Net carb= 0g

▤ Thai Shrimp Salad, low-carb dressing, (7oz (200g)): GI of 35, GL of 2, Net carb= 7g

▤ Thai Squid Salad, low-carb dressing, (7oz (200g)): GI of 40, GL of 2, Net carb= 6g

▤ Tilapia, (3 oz (85g)): GI of 0, GL of 0, Net carb= 0g

▤ Tilefish, (3 oz (85g)): GI of 0, GL of 0, Net carb= 0g

▤ Triggerfish, (3 oz (85g)): GI of 0, GL of 0, Net carb= 0g

▤ Trout, (3 oz (85g)): GI of 0, GL of 0, Net carb= 0g

▤ Tuna, (3 oz (85g)): GI of 0, GL of 0, Net carb= 0g

▤ Tuna and White Bean Salad, low-carb dressing, (7oz (200g)): GI of 35, GL of 2, Net carb= 6g

▤ Tuna Nicoise Salad, low-carb dressing, (8oz (250g)): GI of 50, GL of 5, Net carb= 10g

▤ Tuna Pasta Salad, low-carb dressing, (7oz (200g)): GI of 45, GL of 4, Net carb= 9g

▤ Wahoo, (3 oz (85g)): GI of 0, GL of 0, Net carb= 0g

▤ White Bass, (3 oz (85g)): GI of 0, GL of 0, Net carb= 0g

▤ White Perch, (3 oz (85g)): GI of 0, GL of 0, Net carb= 0g

▤ Whitefish, (3 oz (85g)): GI of 0, GL of 0, Net carb= 0g

▤ Wrasse, (3 oz (85g)): GI of 0, GL of 0, Net carb= 0g

▤ Yellowfin Tuna, (3 oz (85g)): GI of 0, GL of 0, Net carb= 0g

▤ Yellowtail, (3 oz (85g)): GI of 0, GL of 0, Net carb= 0g

▤ Yellowtail Amberjack, (3 oz (85g)): GI of 0, GL of 0, Net carb= 0g

FRUITS AND FRUITS PRODUCTS

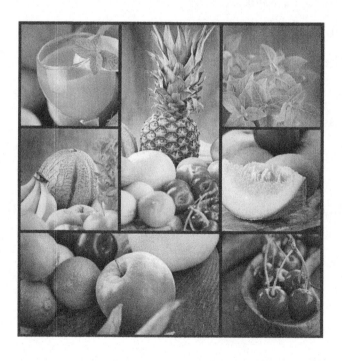

Fruits, with their spectrum of colors and flavors, hold a special place in balanced diets, offering abundant source of vitamins, minerals, and fiber. For those on the DiabeteBalance Diet, navigating the world of fruits and fruit products is crucial. Not all fruits have the same impact on blood sugar. Whole fruits, with their natural sugars balanced by fiber, are usually a healthy choice. However, fruit products, like juices and processed snacks, might lack the fiber and can sometimes contain added sugars, impacting blood sugar levels differently. Being mindful of the type and form of fruit, as well as its preparation, allows individuals to harness the nutritional benefits while managing their diabetes effectively. By appreciating the nuances of fruits and their products, one can integrate them wisely into a dietary regimen, promoting both diabetes management and holistic health.

Benefits of Fruits and Fruit Products:

- **Rich in Nutrients:** Fruits are abundant in essential nutrients like vitamins, minerals, trace minerals, and dietary fiber, contributing to general health and wellness.
- **Low in Fat and Calories:** Most fruits are low in fat and calories, aligning with weight management goals.
- **High in Fiber:** The dietary fiber in fruits helps in controlling sugar absorption into the bloodstream, preventing sudden spikes in glucose and insulin levels.

Potential Drawbacks:

- **Sugar Content:** Some fruits and fruit products, especially processed ones, may contain high natural and added sugar levels, causing potential blood glucose spikes.
- **Processed Fruit Products:** Items like canned fruits, fruit juices, and dried fruits often contain added sugars and have reduced fiber content, making them less ideal for diabetes management.

Guidelines for Incorporating Fruits and Fruit Products:

- **Choose Whole Fruits:** Whole fruits are generally more

beneficial than processed versions, with higher fiber content and fewer added sugars.
- **Monitor Portion Sizes:** Though nutritious, fruits contain carbohydrates and sugars; hence, portion control is key.
- **Read Labels Diligently:** When purchasing fruit products, scrutinize labels for added sugars and high fiber content, favoring those that align with dietary goals.

Comprehensive Selection for the DiabeteBalance Diet:

Below, you'll find an alphabetical list of foods in harmony with the DiabeteBalance Diet. The details on serving size, Glycemic Index (GI), Glycemic Load (GL), and Net Carbohydrates are provided to equip you with essential knowledge for informed portion control and meal planning.

LOW GLYCEMIC LOAD FOODS A-Z

Acai, (½ cup (100g) pulp): GI of 40, GL of 2, Net carb= 5g

Abiyuch, (½ cup (64g)): GI of 45, GL of 7.2, Net carb= 16g

Acerola, (1 cup (98g)): GI of 25, GL of 2, Net carb= 8g

Acerola Juice, (½ cup (120ml)): GI of 30-40, GL of 2.4, Net carb= 6g

Ackee, (½ cup (100g)): GI of 50, GL of 4, Net carb= 8g

African Cherry Orange, (1 fruit (40g)): GI of 40, GL of 2, Net carb= 4g

African Cucumber, (½ cup (60g)): GI of 40, GL of 2, Net carb= 4g

Apple, (1 medium (182g)): GI of 36, GL of 5, Net carb= 21g

Apple Baked Unsweetened, (1 cup (125g)): GI of 35-40, GL of 8, Net carb= 23g

▤ Apple Butter, (1 tbsp (20g)): GI of 40-45, GL of 6, Net carb= 10g

▤ Apple Chips, (1 cup (30g)): GI of 45-50, GL of 10, Net carb= 22g

▤ Apple Juice, (½ cup (120ml)): GI of 45, GL of 6.3, Net carb= 14g

▤ Apple Juice Concentrate, (¼ cup (60g)): GI of 40, GL of 12, Net carb= 15g

▤ Apple Pickled, (½ cup (75g)): GI of 30-35, GL of 4, Net carb= 12g

▤ Applesauce, Canned Light Syrup Drained, (¼ cup (61g)): GI of 40, GL of 5, Net carb= 12.5g

▤ Apricot, (1 fruit (35g)): GI of 34, GL of 2, Net carb= 4g

▤ Apricot Jam, (1 tbsp (20g)): GI of 50-55, GL of 8, Net carb= 13g

▤ Apricot Juice Concentrate, (¼ cup (60g)): GI of 40, GL of 6, Net carb= 12g

▤ Apricot Plum, (1 fruit (50g)): GI of 34, GL of 2, Net carb= 7g

▤ Apricots, Canned Light Syrup Drained, (½ cup (122g)): GI of 40-45, GL of 7, Net carb= 14g

▤ Asian Pears, (1 medium (166g)): GI of 30-35, GL of 6, Net carb= 17g

▤ Avocado, (½ medium (100g)): GI of 15, GL of 0.3, Net carb= 2g

▤ Babaco, (½ cup (75g)): GI of 30, GL of 2, Net carb= 5g

▤ Banana Passionfruit, (1 fruit (20g)): GI of 35, GL of 1, Net carb= 3g

▤ Barbados Cherry, (½ cup (75g)): GI of 30, GL of 2, Net carb= 6g

▤ Bartlett Pears, (1 medium (166g)): GI of 30-35, GL of 6, Net carb= 20g

▤ Beet Juice, (½ cup (120ml)): GI of 64, GL of 5, Net carb= 11g

▤ Black Sapote, (½ cup (50g)): GI of 35, GL of 3, Net carb= 9g

▤ Blackberries, (1 cup (144g)): GI of 25-30, GL of 3, Net carb= 10g

▤ Blackberries, Canned Light Syrup Drained, (½ cup (122g)): GI of 25, GL of 3, Net carb= 8g

▤ Blackberry, (½ cup (72g)): GI of 25, GL of 2, Net carb= 7g

▤ Blackberry Jam, (1 tbsp (20g)): GI of 50-55, GL of 8, Net carb= 13g

▤ Blackcurrant Juice Concentrate, (¼ cup (60g)): GI of 20, GL of 0, Net carb= 0g

▤ Blueberries, (1 cup (148g)): GI of 40-45, GL of 6, Net carb= 17g

▤ Blueberries Canned Light Syrup Drained, (1 cup (230g)): GI of 40-45, GL of 10, Net carb= 23g

▤ Blueberries, Canned Light Syrup Drained, (½ cup (122g)): GI of 40, GL of 7, Net carb= 15g

▤ Blueberry, (½ cup (75g)): GI of 40, GL of 4, Net carb= 10g

▤ Blueberry Jam, (1 tbsp (20g)): GI of 50-55, GL of 8, Net carb= 13g

▤ Blueberry Juice, (½ cup (120ml)): GI of 40, GL of 5.8, Net carb= 14g

▤ Blueberry Juice Concentrate, (¼ cup (60g)): GI of 55, GL of 6.3, Net carb= 12g

▤ Boysenberries, (1 cup (144g)): GI of 25-30, GL of 4, Net carb= 12g

▤ Boysenberry, (½ cup (75g)): GI of 30, GL of 3, Net carb= 8g

▤ Breadfruit, (½ cup (60g)): GI of 60, GL of 6, Net carb= 12g

▤ California Avocados, (½ avocado (100g)): GI of 15-20, GL of 1, Net carb= 3g

▤ California Grapefruit, (1 medium (154g)): GI of 25-30, GL of 4, Net carb= 13g

▤ California Valencia Oranges, (1 medium (131g)): GI of 40-45, GL of 6, Net carb= 14g

- Cantaloupe, (½ cup (89g)): GI of 60, GL of 4, Net carb= 7g

- Cape Gooseberry, (½ cup (50g)): GI of 40, GL of 3, Net carb= 7g

- Carambola (starfruit), (1 fruit (92g)): GI of 30, GL of 2, Net carb= 6g

- Carissa, (1 cup (132g)): GI of 35-40, GL of 7, Net carb= 18g

- Carrot Juice, (½ cup (120ml)): GI of 43, GL of 4.1, Net carb= 9.5g

- Casaba Melon, (1 cup (160g)): GI of 30-35, GL of 4, Net carb= 11g

- Cempedak, (½ cup (75g)): GI of 40, GL of 4, Net carb= 10g

- Cherimoya, (½ fruit (85g)): GI of 35, GL of 3, Net carb= 9g

- Cherries, Canned Light Syrup Drained, (½ cup (122g)): GI of 55-60, GL of 9, Net carb= 18g

- Cherry, (½ cup (76g)): GI of 22, GL of 3, Net carb= 10g

- Cherry Juice, (½ cup (120ml)): GI of 50, GL of 7, Net carb= 14g

- Cherry Preserves, (1 tbsp (20g)): GI of 50-55, GL of 8, Net carb= 13g

- Chokeberry, (½ cup (60g)): GI of 35, GL of 2, Net carb= 6g

- Clementine, (1 fruit (74g)): GI of 35, GL of 3, Net carb= 9g

- Cloudberry, (½ cup (60g)): GI of 25, GL of 2, Net carb= 5g

- Coconut, (½ cup (40g) shredded): GI of 45, GL of 2, Net carb= 5g

- Cornelian Cherry, (½ cup (75g)): GI of 30, GL of 2, Net carb= 6g

- Cranberry, (½ cup (50g)): GI of 45, GL of 3, Net carb= 6g

- Cranberry Juice, (½ cup (120ml)): GI of 52, GL of 7.5, Net carb= 15g

- Cranberry Juice Concentrate, (¼ cup (60g)): GI of 50, GL of 5, Net carb= 10g

▤ Cranberry Sauce, (1 tbsp (20g)): GI of 50-55, GL of 8, Net carb= 13g

▤ Currant, (½ cup (56g)): GI of 25, GL of 2, Net carb= 8g

▤ Damson, (½ cup (75g)): GI of 30, GL of 3, Net carb= 8g

▤ Date, (¼ cup (30g)): GI of 42, GL of 10, Net carb= 24g

▤ Date Plum, (1 fruit (25g)): GI of 35, GL of 2, Net carb= 5g

▤ Desert Lime, (1 fruit (30g)): GI of 30, GL of 1, Net carb= 3g

▤ Dragonfruit, (½ fruit (100g)): GI of 30, GL of 2, Net carb= 6g

▤ Dried Apple, (¼ cup (28g)): GI of 44, GL of 10, Net carb= 16g

▤ Dried Coconut, (¼ cup (20g)): GI of 40, GL of 3, Net carb= 7g

▤ Dried Dragon Fruit, (¼ cup (28g)): GI of 55, GL of 9, Net carb= 15g

▤ Dried Goji Berries, (¼ cup (28g)): GI of 29, GL of 7, Net carb= 14g

▤ Dried Guava, (¼ cup (30g)): GI of 45, GL of 10, Net carb= 18g

▤ Dried Peach, (¼ cup (36g)): GI of 35, GL of 10, Net carb= 20g

▤ Dried Raspberries, (¼ cup (30g)): GI of 40, GL of 8, Net carb= 16g

▤ Dried Strawberries, (¼ cup (30g)): GI of 50, GL of 10, Net carb= 18g

▤ Durian, (½ cup (100g)): GI of 45, GL of 6, Net carb= 13g

▤ Elderberry, (½ cup (50g)): GI of 25, GL of 2, Net carb= 6g

▤ Feijoa, (1 fruit (50g)): GI of 35, GL of 2, Net carb= 6g

▤ Fig, (1 medium (50g)): GI of 60, GL of 8, Net carb= 14g

▤ Fig Preserves, (1 tbsp (20g)): GI of 50-55, GL of 8, Net carb= 13g

▤ Finger Lime, (1 fruit (10g)): GI of 30, GL of 0, Net carb= 1g

▤ Fruit cocktail, Canned Light Syrup Drained, (½ cup (122g)): GI of 55, GL of 8, Net carb= 16g

▤ Gac Fruit, (¼ cup (25g) pulp): GI of 30, GL of 1, Net carb= 2g

▤ Galia Melon, (½ cup (90g)): GI of 65, GL of 4, Net carb= 6g

▤ Genip, (1 fruit (20g)): GI of 35, GL of 1, Net carb= 3g

▤ Goji Berries Dried, (¼ cup (28g)): GI of 35-40, GL of 5, Net carb= 12g

▤ Golden Delicious Apples, (1 medium (174g)): GI of 35-40, GL of 6, Net carb= 17g

▤ Goldenberry, (½ cup (50g)): GI of 35, GL of 3, Net carb= 6g

▤ Gooseberry, (½ cup (75g)): GI of 25, GL of 2, Net carb= 8g

▤ Granny Smith Apples, (1 medium (170g)): GI of 30-35, GL of 5, Net carb= 14g

▤ Grape, (½ cup (75g)): GI of 46, GL of 5, Net carb= 13g

▤ Grape Jelly, (1 tbsp (20g)): GI of 50-55, GL of 8, Net carb= 13g

▤ Grapefruit, (1 medium (154g)): GI of 25-30, GL of 4, Net carb= 13g

▤ Grapefruit Juice, (½ cup (120ml)): GI of 48, GL of 5, Net carb= 11g

▤ Grapefruit segments, Canned Light Syrup Drained, (½ cup (122g)): GI of 25, GL of 3, Net carb= 10g

▤ Grapes, (½ cup (76g)): GI of 45-50, GL of 4, Net carb= 9g

▤ Graviola (Soursop), (½ cup (100g) pulp): GI of 40, GL of 4, Net carb= 10g

▤ Greengage, (1 fruit (20g)): GI of 30, GL of 1, Net carb= 3g

▤ Groundcherries, (1 cup (140g)): GI of 35-40, GL of 7, Net carb= 20g

▤ Guanabana, (½ cup (100g) pulp): GI of 40, GL of 4, Net carb= 10g

▤ Guava, (1 medium (55g)): GI of 20, GL of 1, Net carb= 4g

▤ Guava Juice, (½ cup (120ml)): GI of 33, GL of 3.3, Net carb= 10g

▤ Guava, Canned Light Syrup Drained, (½ cup (122g)): GI of 35-50, GL of 5, Net carb= 10g

▤ Hala Fruit, (¼ cup (25g) pulp): GI of 35, GL of 1, Net carb= 2g

▤ Honeydew Melon, (½ cup (85g)): GI of 60, GL of 4, Net carb= 8g

▤ Huckleberry, (½ cup (75g)): GI of 25, GL of 2, Net carb= 6g

▤ Imbe, (1 fruit (20g)): GI of 40, GL of 1, Net carb= 2g

▤ Jabuticaba, (½ cup (50g)): GI of 35, GL of 3, Net carb= 6g

▤ Jackfruit, (½ cup (100g)): GI of 50, GL of 8, Net carb= 16g

▤ Jambul, (½ cup (75g)): GI of 30, GL of 2, Net carb= 5g

▤ Japanese Plum, (1 fruit (40g)): GI of 40, GL of 2, Net carb= 4g

▤ Jujube, (1 fruit (15g)): GI of 50, GL of 3, Net carb= 6g

▤ Jumbo Olives, (¼ cup (40g)): GI of 45214, GL of 0, Net carb= 1g

▤ Kaffir Lime, (1 fruit (30g)): GI of 30, GL of 1, Net carb= 2g

▤ Kei Apple, (1 fruit (20g)): GI of 35, GL of 1, Net carb= 3g

▤ Kitembilla, (½ cup (50g)): GI of 30, GL of 2, Net carb= 5g

▤ Kiwano (Horned Melon), (½ fruit (100g)): GI of 35, GL of 2, Net carb= 7g

▤ Kiwi, (1 fruit (69g)): GI of 50, GL of 5, Net carb= 9g

▤ Kumquat, (5 fruits (50g)): GI of 30, GL of 3, Net carb= 6g

▤ Langsat, (½ cup (75g)): GI of 40, GL of 3, Net carb= 8g

▤ Lemon, (1 fruit (58g)): GI of 20, GL of 1, Net carb= 3g

▤ Lemon Curd, (1 tbsp (20g)): GI of 50-55, GL of 8, Net carb= 13g

▤ Lemon Juice, (½ cup (120ml)): GI of 20, GL of 2, Net carb= 10.5g

▤ Lemon Juice Concentrate, (1 tbsp (15g)): GI of 20, GL of 0.2, Net carb= 1g

▤ Lime, (1 fruit (44g)): GI of 20, GL of 1, Net carb= 3g

▤ Lime Juice Concentrate, (1 tbsp (15g)): GI of 20, GL of 0.2, Net carb= 1g

▤ Limequat, (1 fruit (20g)): GI of 30, GL of 1, Net carb= 2g

▤ Loganberries, (1 cup (180g)): GI of 25-30, GL of 3, Net carb= 9g

▤ Longan, (½ cup (50g)): GI of 50, GL of 5, Net carb= 10g

▤ Loquat, (½ cup (75g)): GI of 35, GL of 2, Net carb= 5g

▤ Lychee, (½ cup (75g)): GI of 50, GL of 6, Net carb= 12g

▤ Mandarin Orange, (1 fruit (88g)): GI of 40, GL of 4, Net carb= 9g

▤ Mandarin oranges, Canned Light Syrup Drained, (½ cup (122g)): GI of 45, GL of 6, Net carb= 13g

▤ Mango, (½ cup (83g)): GI of 55, GL of 8, Net carb= 15g

▤ Mango Jam, (1 tbsp (20g)): GI of 50-55, GL of 8, Net carb= 13g

▤ Mango Juice, (½ cup (120ml)): GI of 41, GL of 6.2, Net carb= 15g

▤ Mango Pickled, (¼ cup (60g)): GI of 40-45, GL of 6, Net carb= 12g

▤ Mango, Canned Light Syrup Drained, (½ cup (122g)): GI of 40-50, GL of 8, Net carb= 16g

▤ Mangosteen, (1 fruit (75g)): GI of 45, GL of 3, Net carb= 6g

▤ Marula, (1 fruit (10g)): GI of 30, GL of 1, Net carb= 1g

▤ Medlar, (1 fruit (20g)): GI of 35, GL of 1, Net carb= 3g

▤ Melon, (1 cup (177g)): GI of 65, GL of 5, Net carb= 12g

▤ Miracle Fruit, (1 fruit (5g)): GI of 30, GL of 0, Net carb= 1g

▤ Mixed Berry Jam, (1 tbsp (20g)): GI of 50-55, GL of 8, Net carb= 13g

▤ Mulberry, (½ cup (70g)): GI of 25, GL of 3, Net carb= 6g

▤ Nagami Kumquat, (5 fruits (50g)): GI of 30, GL of 3, Net carb= 6g

▤ Nance, (1 cup (120g)): GI of 40-45, GL of 10, Net carb= 20g

▤ Navel Oranges, (1 medium (154g)): GI of 35-40, GL of 6, Net carb= 15g

▤ Nectarine, (1 medium (142g)): GI of 40, GL of 4, Net carb= 11g

▤ Nectarines, (1 medium (142g)): GI of 35-40, GL of 6, Net carb= 15g

▤ Oheloberries, (1 cup (140g)): GI of 30-35, GL of 5, Net carb= 11g

▤ Okra Pickled, (1 cup (160g)): GI of 15-20, GL of 1, Net carb= 3g

▤ Olive, (5 large (25g)): GI of 15, GL of 0, Net carb= 1g

▤ Orange, (1 medium (131g)): GI of 40, GL of 4, Net carb= 12g

▤ Orange Juice, (½ cup (120ml)): GI of 50, GL of 6.5, Net carb= 13g

▤ Orange Marmalade, (1 tbsp (20g)): GI of 50-55, GL of 8, Net carb= 13g

▤ Papaya, (1 cup (145g)): GI of 60, GL of 6, Net carb= 11g

▤ Papaya, Canned Light Syrup Drained, (½ cup (122g)): GI of 55-60, GL of 7, Net carb= 14g

▤ Passion Fruit, (1 fruit (18g)): GI of 30, GL of 1, Net carb= 2g

▤ Passionfruit Juice, (½ cup (120ml)): GI of 30, GL of 2.1, Net carb= 7g

▤ Passionfruit Juice Concentrate, (¼ cup (60g)): GI of 35, GL of 3, Net carb= 8.7g

▤ Pawpaw, (1 cup (140g)): GI of 60, GL of 6, Net carb= 11g

▤ Peach, (1 medium (150g)): GI of 40, GL of 4, Net carb= 10g

▤ Peach Juice, (½ cup (120ml)): GI of 42, GL of 6, Net carb= 14g

▤ Peach Juice Concentrate, (¼ cup (60g)): GI of 40, GL of 6, Net carb= 12g

▤ Peach Pickled, (½ cup (130g)): GI of 40-45, GL of 8, Net carb= 16g

▤ Peach Preserves, (1 tbsp (20g)): GI of 50-55, GL of 8, Net carb= 13g

▤ Peaches, Canned Light Syrup Drained, (½ cup (122g)): GI of 40-45, GL of 8, Net carb= 16g

▤ Pear, (1 medium (178g)): GI of 38, GL of 5, Net carb= 21g

▤ Pear Juice, (½ cup (120ml)): GI of 44, GL of 5.5, Net carb= 14g

▤ Pears Canned Extra Light Syrup, (½ cup (122g)): GI of 40-45, GL of 5.5, Net carb= 11g

▤ Pears, Canned Light Syrup Drained, (½ cup (122g)): GI of 43, GL of 7, Net carb= 15g

▤ Peppers Pickled, (1 cup (150g)): GI of 15-20, GL of 1, Net carb= 3g

▤ Persimmon, (1 fruit (25g)): GI of 50, GL of 3, Net carb= 6g

▤ Pineapple, (½ cup (82g)): GI of 59, GL of 7, Net carb= 10g

▤ Pineapple Juice, (½ cup (120ml)): GI of 46, GL of 6.5, Net carb= 14g

▤ Pineapple Preserves, (1 tbsp (20g)): GI of 50-55, GL of 8, Net carb= 13g

▤ Pineapple, Canned Extra Light Syrup, (½ cup (122g)): GI of 50-55, GL of 7.5, Net carb= 15g

▤ Pitanga, (1 cup (140g)): GI of 35-40, GL of 7, Net carb= 14g

▤ Plum, (1 fruit (66g)): GI of 40, GL of 2, Net carb= 6g

▤ Plum Jam, (1 tbsp (20g)): GI of 50-55, GL of 8, Net carb= 13g

▤ Plum Pickled, (1 cup (150g)): GI of 30-35, GL of 6, Net carb= 12g

▤ Plums Canned Extra Purple Light Syrup, (½ cup (122g)): GI of 40-45, GL of 6.7, Net carb= 15g

▤ Plums, Canned Light Syrup Drained, (½ cup (122g)): GI of 40, GL of 6, Net carb= 12g

▤ Pomegranate, (½ cup (87g)): GI of 53, GL of 6, Net carb= 12g

▤ Pomegranate Juice, (½ cup (120ml)): GI of 53, GL of 9, Net carb= 17g

▤ Pomegranate Juice Concentrate, (¼ cup (60g)): GI of 35, GL of 8, Net carb= 12g

▤ Pomelo, (½ fruit (154g)): GI of 30, GL of 3, Net carb= 9g

▤ Prickly Pear, (1 fruit (103g)): GI of 35, GL of 2, Net carb= 5g

▤ Prunes, (¼ cup (40g)): GI of 29, GL of 10, Net carb= 18g

▤ Pummelo, (1 cup sections (190g)): GI of 30-35, GL of 4, Net carb= 8g

▤ Purple Passion Fruit Juice, (½ cup (120ml)): GI of 30-35, GL of 5, Net carb= 10g

▤ Quince, (1 fruit (92g)): GI of 34, GL of 2, Net carb= 6g

▤ Quince Jelly, (1 tbsp (20g)): GI of 50-55, GL of 8, Net carb= 13g

▤ Raspberries, Canned Light Syrup Drained, (½ cup (122g)): GI of 32, GL of 3, Net carb= 9g

▤ Raspberry, (½ cup (62g)): GI of 32, GL of 1, Net carb= 3g

▤ Raspberry Jam, (1 tbsp (20g)): GI of 50-55, GL of 8, Net carb= 13g

▤ Raspberry Juice Concentrate, (¼ cup (60g)): GI of 40, GL of 5, Net carb= 10g

▤ Red Banana, (1 medium (100g)): GI of 45, GL of 7, Net carb= 18g

▤ Red Currant Jelly, (1 tbsp (20g)): GI of 50-55, GL of 8, Net carb= 13g

▤ Redcurrant, (½ cup (56g)): GI of 25, GL of 2, Net carb= 5g

▤ Rhubarb, (1 cup (122g)): GI of 15, GL of 1, Net carb= 3g

▤ Rose Apple, (1 fruit (45g)): GI of 30, GL of 1, Net carb= 3g

▤ Santa Claus Melon, (1 cup (177g)): GI of 60, GL of 6, Net carb= 13g

▤ Sapodilla, (1 fruit (150g)): GI of 45, GL of 6, Net carb= 14g

▤ Soursop, (1 cup (225g)): GI of 45, GL of 6, Net carb= 15g

▤ Star Apple, (1 fruit (138g)): GI of 35, GL of 3, Net carb= 6g

▤ Star Fruit, (1 fruit (91g)): GI of 25, GL of 1, Net carb= 4g

▤ Strawberries, Canned Light Syrup Drained, (½ cup (122g)): GI of 40, GL of 4, Net carb= 10g

▤ Strawberry, (½ cup (72g)): GI of 32, GL of 1, Net carb= 4g

▤ Strawberry Jam, (1 tbsp (20g)): GI of 50-55, GL of 8, Net carb= 13g

▤ Strawberry Juice Concentrate, (¼ cup (60g)): GI of 40, GL of 5, Net carb= 10g

▤ Sweet Granadilla, (1 fruit (140g)): GI of 40, GL of 3, Net carb= 10g

▤ Tahitian Pomelo, (½ fruit (154g)): GI of 40, GL of 4, Net carb= 10g

▤ Tamarind, (1 oz (28g)): GI of 40, GL of 3, Net carb= 6g

▤ Tangelo, (1 fruit (109g)): GI of 42, GL of 4, Net carb= 10g

▤ Tangerine, (1 fruit (84g)): GI of 40, GL of 3, Net carb= 9g

▤ Tomato Juice, (1 cup (240ml)): GI of 38, GL of 3.8, Net carb= 10g

▤ Tsukemono Japanese Pickles, (1 cup (150g)): GI of 15-20, GL of 2, Net carb= 4g

▤ Turnip Pickled, (1 cup (150g)): GI of 15-20, GL of 1, Net carb= 3g

- Ugli Fruit, (½ fruit (120g)): GI of 40, GL of 4, Net carb= 10g
- Ugni Fruit, (¼ cup (30g)): GI of 30, GL of 2, Net carb= 4g
- Vanilla Bean, (1 bean (6g)): GI of 50, GL of 1, Net carb= 1g
- Velvet Apple, (1 fruit (166g)): GI of 35, GL of 3, Net carb= 9g
- Wampi, (¼ cup (28g)): GI of 30, GL of 1, Net carb= 3g
- Watermelon, (1 cup (152g)): GI of 72, GL of 5, Net carb= 11g
- Watermelon Juice, (½ cup (120ml)): GI of 72, GL of 7.2, Net carb= 9g
- White Currant, (½ cup (56g)): GI of 25, GL of 2, Net carb= 5g
- White Sapote, (1 fruit (170g)): GI of 30, GL of 2, Net carb= 6g
- Yellow Passion Fruit, (1 fruit (18g)): GI of 30, GL of 1, Net carb= 2g
- Yellow Watermelon, (1 cup (152g)): GI of 72, GL of 5, Net carb= 11g
- Yuzu, (1 fruit (77g)): GI of 30, GL of 1, Net carb= 2g
- Zante Currant, (¼ cup (40g)): GI of 60, GL of 10, Net carb= 17g
- Ziziphus Fruit, (1 fruit (10g)): GI of 35, GL of 1, Net carb= 3g
- Zombie Fruit (a type of passion fruit), (1 fruit (18g)): GI of 30, GL of 1, Net carb= 2g
- Zucchini Squash, (1 cup (124g)): GI of 15, GL of 1, Net carb= 3g
- Zwetschge (a type of plum), (1 fruit (66g)): GI of 40, GL of 2, Net carb= 5g

MEDIUM GLYCEMIC LOAD FOODS A-Z

In the DiabeteBalance Diet, we prioritize a strategic approach that empowers you to make informed dietary choices. While we empha-size foods with a low glycemic load as the adequate choice for opti-mally managing type 2 diabetes, we understand the need for variety and occasional indulgences.

Thus, we also provide comprehensive information on foods that fall within the medium glycemic load category. These are not the optimal option for regular consumption, but we believe in giving you a complete understanding of your options to help you navigate your food choices.

For each food item in this medium category, we present key details including typical serving size, Glycemic Index (GI), Glycemic Load (GL), and Net Carbohydrates. Armed with this information, you can make more conscious decisions even when you decide to consume these foods on occasion.

However, it's crucial to remember that portion control is vital when indulging in these foods. While they can be tolerated occasionally, we highly recommend reducing the standard serving size to ensure that your intake stays below 15 grams of net carbohydrates. This approach will help you maintain better blood sugar control while still allowing some flexibility in your diet.

≣ Ambrosia, (½ cup (120g)): GI of 54, GL of 10.8, Net carb= 20g

≣ Banana, (1 extra small (105g)): GI of 51-65, GL of 15.6, Net carb= 24g

≣ Banana Baked, (1 extra small (105g)): GI of 60-60, GL of 19.3, Net carb= 28g

≣ Dates, (¼cup (40g)): GI of 42, GL of 18, Net carb= 28g

≣ Dried Apricots, Unsweetened, (¼ cup (32g)): GI of 32, GL of 12, Net carb= 18g

≣ Dried Banana, Unsweetened, (¼cup (30g)): GI of 54, GL of 14, Net carb= 22g

▤ Dried Blueberries, Unsweetened, (¼ cup (40g)): GI of 53, GL of 14, Net carb= 26g

▤ Dried Cherries, Unsweetened, (¼ cup (40g)): GI of 54, GL of 16, Net carb= 30g

▤ Dried Cranberries, Unsweetened, (¼ cup (40g)): GI of 64, GL of 18, Net carb= 28g

▤ Dried Currants, Unsweetened, (¼ cup (40g)): GI of 56, GL of 17, Net carb= 30g

▤ Dried Custard Apple, Unsweetened, (¼ cup (30g)): GI of 48, GL of 13, Net carb= 22g

▤ Dried Kiwi, Unsweetened, (¼ cup (30g)): GI of 54, GL of 11, Net carb= 19g

▤ Dried Longan, Unsweetened, (¼ cup (32g)): GI of 55, GL of 15, Net carb= 28g

▤ Dried Lychee, Unsweetened, (¼ cup (30g)): GI of 52, GL of 13, Net carb= 22g

▤ Dried Mango, Unsweetened, (¼ cup (30g)): GI of 55, GL of 12, Net carb= 22g

▤ Dried Papaya, Unsweetened, (¼ cup (30g)): GI of 60, GL of 15, Net carb= 25g

▤ Dried Pear, Unsweetened, (¼ cup (40g)): GI of 43, GL of 12, Net carb= 24g

▤ Dried Persimmon, Unsweetened, (¼ cup (32g)): GI of 53, GL of 15, Net carb= 24g

▤ Dried Pineapple, Unsweetened, (¼ cup (35g)): GI of 58, GL of 16, Net carb= 28g

▤ Dried Sapodilla, Unsweetened, (¼ cup (30g)): GI of 50, GL of 12, Net carb= 20g

▤ Figs, (¼ cup (40g)): GI of 61, GL of 15, Net carb= 24g

▤ Golden Seedless Raisins, (¼ cup (40g)): GI of 50-55, GL of 17, Net carb= 31g

▤ Grape Juice Concentrate, (¼ cup (60g)): GI of 70, GL of 12, Net carb= 15g

▤ Guava Nectar Canned, (1 cup (240g)): GI of 40-45, GL of 15, Net carb= 30g

▤ Guava Sauce Cooked, (1 cup (250g)): GI of 40-45, GL of 14, Net carb= 28g

▤ Litchis, (1 cup (190g)): GI of 50-55, GL of 14, Net carb= 25g

▤ Mango Cooked, (1 cup (165g)): GI of 45-50, GL of 15, Net carb= 30g

▤ Plantain, (1 cup, sliced (148g)): GI of 40, GL of 12, Net carb= 30g

▤ Prune Puree, (¼ cup (60g)): GI of 40-45, GL of 12, Net carb= 24g

▤ Prune Whip, (1/2 cup (125g)): GI of 40-45, GL of 14, Net carb= 28g

---

MEDIUM GLYCEMIC LOAD FOODS A-Z

Consider reducing the serving size to stay below 15 grams of net carbs

▤ Ambrosia, (½ cup (120g)): GI of 54, GL of 10.8, Net carb= 20g

▤ Banana, (1 extra small (105g)): GI of 51-65, GL of 15.6, Net carb= 24g

▤ Banana Baked, (1 extra small (105g)): GI of 60-60, GL of 19.3, Net carb= 28g

▤ Dates, (¼cup (40g)): GI of 42, GL of 18, Net carb= 28g

▤ Dried Apricots, Unsweetened, (¼ cup (32g)): GI of 32, GL of 12, Net carb= 18g

▤ Dried Banana, Unsweetened, (¼cup (30g)): GI of 54, GL of 14, Net carb= 22g

▤ Dried Blueberries, Unsweetened, (¼ cup (40g)): GI of 53, GL of 14, Net carb= 26g

▤ Dried Cherries, Unsweetened, (¼ cup (40g)): GI of 54, GL of 16, Net carb= 30g

▤ Dried Cranberries, Unsweetened, (¼ cup (40g)): GI of 64, GL of 18, Net carb= 28g

▤ Dried Currants, Unsweetened, (¼ cup (40g)): GI of 56, GL of 17, Net carb= 30g

▤ Dried Custard Apple, Unsweetened, (¼ cup (30g)): GI of 48, GL of 13, Net carb= 22g

▤ Dried Kiwi, Unsweetened, (¼ cup (30g)): GI of 54, GL of 11, Net carb= 19g

▤ Dried Longan, Unsweetened, (¼ cup (32g)): GI of 55, GL of 15, Net carb= 28g

▤ Dried Lychee, Unsweetened, (¼ cup (30g)): GI of 52, GL of 13, Net carb= 22g

▤ Dried Mango, Unsweetened, (¼ cup (30g)): GI of 55, GL of 12, Net carb= 22g

▤ Dried Papaya, Unsweetened, (¼ cup (30g)): GI of 60, GL of 15, Net carb= 25g

▤ Dried Pear, Unsweetened, (¼ cup (40g)): GI of 43, GL of 12, Net carb= 24g

▤ Dried Persimmon, Unsweetened, (¼ cup (32g)): GI of 53, GL of 15, Net carb= 24g

▤ Dried Pineapple, Unsweetened, (¼ cup (35g)): GI of 58, GL of 16, Net carb= 28g

▤ Dried Sapodilla, Unsweetened, (¼ cup (30g)): GI of 50, GL of 12, Net carb= 20g

▤ Figs, (¼ cup (40g)): GI of 61, GL of 15, Net carb= 24g

▤ Golden Seedless Raisins, (¼ cup (40g)): GI of 50-55, GL of 17, Net carb= 31g

▤ Grape Juice Concentrate, (¼ cup (60g)): GI of 70, GL of 12, Net carb= 15g

▤ Guava Nectar Canned, (1 cup (240g)): GI of 40-45, GL of 15, Net carb= 30g

▤ Guava Sauce Cooked, (1 cup (250g)): GI of 40-45, GL of 14, Net carb= 28g

▤ Litchis, (1 cup (190g)): GI of 50-55, GL of 14, Net carb= 25g

▤ Mango Cooked, (1 cup (165g)): GI of 45-50, GL of 15, Net carb= 30g

▤ Plantain, (1 cup, sliced (148g)): GI of 40, GL of 12, Net carb= 30g

▤ Prune Puree, (¼ cup (60g)): GI of 40-45, GL of 12, Net carb= 24g

▤ Prune Whip, (1/2 cup (125g)): GI of 40-45, GL of 14, Net carb= 28g

LEGUMES AND PULSES

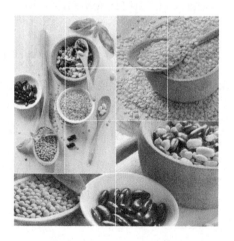

Legumes and pulses offer versatility and nutrition, making them crucial in diabetes management plans. However, their incorporation into the diet requires thoughtful consideration, considering their glycemic load (GL) and compatibility with the DiabeteBalance Diet. By comprehending the advantages and potential challenges of beans and their derivatives, individuals can make informed choices to enhance their diabetes management and overall well-being.

Advantages of legumes and pulses:

- **Rich in Fiber**: Beans and their by-products are renowned for their high fiber content. Dietary fiber moderates the digestion and absorption of carbohydrates, facilitating a gradual release of glucose into the bloodstream. This, in turn, helps avoid abrupt blood sugar spikes, thus enhancing glycemic control.
- **Protein-Heavy**: Beans are a great source of plant-based protein, a vital part of a diabetes-friendly diet. Unlike carbohydrates, protein doesn't significantly affect blood glucose levels and can aid in promoting feelings of fullness, thereby assisting with weight management.
- **Nutrient-Dense**: Beans contain essential nutrients such as iron, magnesium, potassium, and B vitamins. These nutrients support various bodily functions and can counteract the deficiencies often observed in individuals with T2D.

Possible Drawbacks of Beans and By-Products:

- **Digestive Discomfort**: Beans can sometimes lead to digestive discomfort due to their high fiber content. Soaking beans before cooking and chewing them thoroughly can help alleviate these symptoms.
- **Caloric Density**: While beans are nutrient-dense, they are also relatively high in calories. Overconsumption can lead to weight gain, making portion control essential.

Incorporating Beans and By-Products into The DiabeteBalance Diet:

Here are some tips to include beans and their by-products in your diet:

- **Choose Beans as a Protein Source**: Beans can serve as a low-fat, high-fiber alternative to meat or other animal proteins. This substitution can help maintain stable blood sugar levels.

- **Emphasize Whole Foods**: Opt for whole beans over processed bean products to limit sodium and added sugars. Canned beans are acceptable if rinsed thoroughly to remove excess salt.
- **Mind Portion Sizes**: Despite their health benefits, beans are high in calories. Practice portion control to prevent excessive calorie intake. The typical serving size for beans and their by-products is about 15-20 grams. The list provided outline the GL, GI, and net carb content per serving, helping you make an informed choice.
- **Experiment with Bean By-Products**: Consider incorporating by-products such as tofu, tempeh, and edamame into your diet. These provide a protein-rich, low-carb alternative to other protein sources. However, avoid highly processed alternatives such as certain meat substitutes that may be high in additives and sodium.

The following list provides a comprehensive selection of foods that fully comply with the DiabeteBalance Diet. Each entry includes crucial details such as serving size, Glycemic Index (GI), Glycemic Load (GL), and Net Carbohydrates. This information equips you with the knowledge needed to make informed decisions regarding portion sizes and effective meal planning. The foods are sorted alphabetically for easy reference.

▤ Adzuki Bean Flour, (¼ cup, 30g): GI of 32, GL of 5.8, Net carb= 18g

▤ Adzuki Bean Sprout Powder, (¼ cup, 30g): GI of 15, GL of 2.1, Net carb= 14g

▤ Alfalfa Sprout Powder, (¼ cup, 30g): GI of 15, GL of 0.8, Net carb= 5g

▤ Amaranth Sprout Powder, (¼ cup, 30g): GI of 35, GL of 7, Net carb= 20g

▤ Azuki Bean Flour, (¼ cup, 30g): GI of 33, GL of 6.2, Net carb= 18.9g

▤ Baby lima beans, (½ cup, 100g): GI of 32, GL of 6, Net carb= 13g

▤ Barley Sprout Powder, (¼ cup, 30g): GI of 25, GL of 4.5, Net carb= 18g

▤ Black Bean Flour, (¼ cup, 30g): GI of 30, GL of 3.2, Net carb= 10.5g

▤ Black beans, (½ cup, 100g): GI of 30, GL of 5, Net carb= 13g

▤ Black Eyed Pea Flour, (¼ cup, 30g): GI of 42, GL of 7.9, Net carb= 18.9g

▤ Black turtle beans, (½ cup, 100g): GI of 30, GL of 5, Net carb= 13g

▤ Black-eyed peas, (½ cup, 100g): GI of 41, GL of 8, Net carb= 19g

▤ Broad Bean Flour (Fava Bean Flour), (¼ cup, 30g): GI of 79, GL of 13.7, Net carb= 17.4g

▤ Broccoli Sprout Powder, (¼ cup, 30g): GI of 15, GL of 1.2, Net carb= 8g

▤ Buckwheat Sprout Powder, (¼ cup, 30g): GI of 45, GL of 9, Net carb= 20g

▤ Butter Bean Flour (Lima Bean Flour), (¼ cup, 30g): GI of 31, GL of 5.6, Net carb= 18g

▤ Cabbage Sprout Powder, (¼ cup, 30g): GI of 15, GL of 1.2, Net carb= 8g

▤ Cannellini Bean Flour, (¼ cup, 30g): GI of 31, GL of 5.6, Net carb= 18g

▤ Cannellini beans, (½ cup, 100g): GI of 31, GL of 4, Net carb= 13g

▤ Chia Sprout Powder, (¼ cup, 30g): GI of 15, GL of 0.6, Net carb= 4g

▤ Chickpea Flour (Besan), (¼ cup, 30g): GI of 44, GL of 5.8, Net carb= 13.2g

▤ Chickpeas, garbanzo beans, (½ cup, 100g): GI of 28, GL of 6, Net carb= 16g

▤ Clover Sprout Powder, (¼ cup, 30g): GI of 15, GL of 0.8, Net carb= 5g

▤ Cowpeas, (½ cup, 100g): GI of 29, GL of 7, Net carb= 18g

▤ Cranberry Bean Flour, (¼ cup, 30g): GI of 29, GL of 5.2, Net carb= 18g

▤ Dragon's tongue beans, (½ cup, 100g): GI of 31, GL of 2, Net carb= 5g

▤ Fava Bean Flour, (¼ cup, 30g): GI of 79, GL of 13.7, Net carb= 17.4g

▤ Fava beans, (½ cup, 100g): GI of 32, GL of 7, Net carb= 13g

▤ Flageolet beans, (½ cup, 100g): GI of 31, GL of 4, Net carb= 14g

▤ French Green Lentil Flour, (¼ cup, 30g): GI of 28, GL of 5, Net carb= 18g

▤ Garbanzo Bean Flour (Gram Flour), (¼ cup, 30g): GI of 28, GL of 4.9, Net carb= 17.4g

▤ Garlic Sprout Powder, (¼ cup, 30g): GI of 15, GL of 2.1, Net carb= 14g

▤ Great Northern Bean Flour, (¼ cup, 30g): GI of 36, GL of 6.5, Net carb= 18g

▤ Great Northern Beans, (½ cup, 100g): GI of 31, GL of 5, Net carb= 15g

▤ Green Pea Flour, (¼ cup, 30g): GI of 48, GL of 8.6, Net carb= 18g

▤ Green peas, (½ cup, 100g): GI of 68, GL of 4, Net carb= 9g

▤ Kale Sprout Powder, (¼ cup, 30g): GI of 15, GL of 1.2, Net carb= 8g

▤ Kidney Bean Flour, (¼ cup, 30g): GI of 24, GL of 4.3, Net carb= 18g

▤ Kidney beans, (½ cup, 100g): GI of 29, GL of 7, Net carb= 16g

▤ Lentil Flour, (¼ cup, 30g): GI of 29, GL of 4.4, Net carb= 15g

▤ Lentil Sprout Powder, (¼ cup, 30g): GI of 25, GL of 3.8, Net carb= 15g

▤ Lentils, (½ cup, 100g): GI of 29, GL of 5, Net carb= 12g

▤ Lima bean flour, (½ cup, 100g): GI of 32, GL of 4, Net carb= 19g

▤ Lima Bean Flour, (¼ cup, 30g): GI of 32, GL of 5.8, Net carb= 18g

▤ Lima beans, (½ cup, 100g): GI of 32, GL of 8, Net carb= 20g

▤ Moth Bean Flour, (¼ cup, 30g): GI of 29, GL of 5.5, Net carb= 18.9g

▤ Mung Bean Flour, (¼ cup, 30g): GI of 25, GL of 4.7, Net carb= 18.9g

▤ Mung Bean Sprout Powder, (¼ cup, 30g): GI of 15, GL of 1.8, Net carb= 12g

▤ Mung beans, (½ cup, 100g): GI of 32, GL of 4, Net carb= 12g

▤ Navy Bean Flour, (¼ cup, 30g): GI of 38, GL of 6.8, Net carb= 18g

▤ Navy beans, (½ cup, 100g): GI of 31-58, GL of 8, Net carb= 11g

▤ Onion Sprout Powder, (¼ cup, 30g): GI of 15, GL of 2.3, Net carb= 15g

▤ Pea Sprout Powder, (¼ cup, 30g): GI of 15, GL of 2.1, Net carb= 14g

▤ Peanuts, (1 oz, 28g): GI of 30-33, GL of 1, Net carb= 3g

▤ Pinto Bean Flour, (¼ cup, 30g): GI of 39, GL of 7, Net carb= 18g

▤ Quinoa Sprout Powder, (¼ cup, 30g): GI of 35, GL of 7, Net carb= 20g

▤ Radish Sprout Powder, (¼ cup, 30g): GI of 15, GL of 0.8, Net carb= 5g

▤ Red beans, (½ cup, 100g): GI of 35-58, GL of 10, Net carb= 15g

▤ Red kidney beans, (½ cup, 100g): GI of 24-40, GL of 7, Net carb= 13g

▤ Red kidney beans, (½ cup, 100g): GI of 24-40, GL of 7, Net carb= 13g

▤ Red Lentil Flour, (¼ cup, 30g): GI of 26, GL of 4.7, Net carb= 18g

▤ Red Lentil Flour, (¼ cup, 30g): GI of 26, GL of 4.7, Net carb= 18g

▤ Red lentils, (½ cup, 100g): GI of 20-44, GL of 8, Net carb= 13g

▤ Red lentils, (½ cup, 100g): GI of 20-44, GL of 8, Net carb= 13g

▤ Soy Flour, (¼ cup, 30g): GI of 15, GL of 0.9, Net carb= 6g

▤ Soy Flour, (¼ cup, 30g): GI of 15, GL of 0.9, Net carb= 6g

▤ Soybean Sprout Powder, (¼ cup, 30g): GI of 15, GL of 1.2, Net carb= 8g

▤ Soybean Sprout Powder, (¼ cup, 30g): GI of 15, GL of 1.2, Net carb= 8g

▤ Soybeans, (½ cup, 100g): GI of 18-33, GL of 6, Net carb= 10g

▤ Soybeans, (½ cup, 100g): GI of 18-33, GL of 6, Net carb= 10g

▤ Split peas, (½ cup, 100g): GI of 22-32, GL of 5, Net carb= 12g

▤ Split peas, (½ cup, 100g): GI of 22-32, GL of 5, Net carb= 12g

▤ Split peas, (½ cup, 100g): GI of 22-32, GL of 5, Net carb= 12g

▤ Split peas, (½ cup, 100g): GI of 22-32, GL of 5, Net carb= 12g

▤ Sunflower Sprout Powder, (¼ cup, 30g): GI of 15, GL of 1.2, Net carb= 8g

▤ Sunflower Sprout Powder, (¼ cup, 30g): GI of 15, GL of 1.2, Net carb= 8g

▤ Wheatgrass Sprout Powder, (¼ cup, 30g): GI of 15, GL of 2.3, Net carb= 15g

▤ Wheatgrass Sprout Powder, (¼ cup, 30g): GI of 15, GL of 2.3, Net carb= 15g

▤ White Bean Flour, (¼ cup, 30g): GI of 31, GL of 5.6, Net carb= 18g

▤ White beans, (½ cup, 100g): GI of 31-45, GL of 7, Net carb= 12g

▤ Yellow Split Pea Flour, (¼ cup, 30g): GI of 35, GL of 6.3, Net carb= 18g

NUTS AND SEEDS

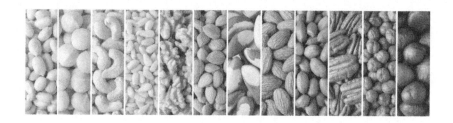

Nuts and seeds are vital in many diets, and they are particularly beneficial for individuals following the DiabeteBalance Diet. Here's a
detailed overview of their potential benefits, drawbacks, and guidelines for incorporation in the diet to manage diabetes effectively.

Benefits of Nuts and Seeds:

- **Nutrient-Rich:** Packed with fiber, protein, healthy fats,
  vitamins, and minerals (e.g., vitamin E, zinc, calcium,
  magnesium,) nuts and seeds contribute to overall health.
- **Blood Sugar Control:** Nuts and seeds promote blood sugar

control thanks to their high fiber and protein content, which supports a gradual release of glucose into the bloodstream and helps with blood sugar regulation.

- **Heart Health:** Nuts and seeds contribute to heart health by raising good HDL cholesterol and reducing bad LDL cholesterol, thereby decreasing the likelihood of heart disease.
- **Antioxidant Content:** High in antioxidants, nuts and seeds combat oxidative stress, helping in cellular damage prevention and inflammation reduction.
- **Protein-Rich:** As a source of plant-based protein, nuts and seeds promote satiety, aiding in weight management, vital for diabetes reversal.

Potential Drawbacks of Nuts and Seeds:

- **High in Calories:** While nutrient-dense, nuts and seeds are calorie-rich, so moderation is key to avoid weight gain.
- **Salted or Coated Varieties:** Avoid commercially prepared nuts and seeds with added sugars, oils, or excessive sodium.

Incorporating Nuts and Seeds into the DiabeteBalance Diet:

- **Choose Raw or Dry-Roasted:** These forms usually lack unhealthy additives.
- **Monitor Portion Sizes:** Mind the high-calorie content; a handful is often an adequate serving.
- **Ideal for Snacks:** Their nutritional profile makes them excellent for managing hunger between meals.
- **Include Nut and Seed Butter:** Nut and seed butter can add versatility to the diet.
- **Versatile Addition:** Use nuts and seeds to enhance salads, oatmeal, yogurt, or stir-fries.

Comprehensive Selection for the DiabeteBalance Diet:

Below is an alphabetical list of nuts and seeds compliant with the DiabeteBalance Diet, complete with serving size, Glycemic Index (GI), Glycemic Load (GL), and Net Carbohydrates. This information supports making well-informed decisions on portion sizes and meal planning.

▤ Almond Butter, (2 tbsp (32g)): GI of 10, GL of 0.3, Net carb= 3g

▤ Almonds, (1 oz (28g)): GI of 7, GL of 1.4, Net carb= 2g

▤ Boiled Chestnuts, (1 oz (28g)): GI of 60, GL of 2, Net carb= 14g

▤ Brazil Nut Butter, (2 tbsp (32g)): GI of 15, GL of 1, Net carb= 2g

▤ Brazil nuts, (1 oz (28g)): GI of 15, GL of 0.2, Net carb= 1g

▤ Butternuts, (1 oz (28g)): GI of 15, GL of 0.3, Net carb= 2g

▤ Cashew Butter, (2 tbsp (32g)): GI of 25, GL of 3, Net carb= 6g

▤ Cashews, (1 oz (28g)): GI of 25, GL of 6, Net carb= 8g

▤ Chestnuts, (1 oz (28g)): GI of 60, GL of 2, Net carb= 14g

▤ Chia Nut Butter, (2 tbsp (32g)): GI of 1, GL of 1, Net carb= 2g

▤ Chia nuts, (1 oz (28g)): GI of 1, GL of 1, Net carb= 1g

▤ Chia seeds, (1 oz (28g)): GI of 1, GL of 1, Net carb= 2g

▤ Coconut, (1 oz (28g)): GI of 51, GL of 6, Net carb= 6g

▤ Fennel seeds, (1 oz (28g)): GI of 5, GL of 1, Net carb= 2g

▤ Fenugreek seeds, (1 oz (28g)): GI of 15, GL of 1, Net carb= 6g

▤ Filbert (Hazelnut) Butter, (2 tbsp (32g)): GI of 0, GL of 0, Net carb= 3g

▤ Filberts (Hazelnuts), (1 oz (28g)): GI of 0, GL of 0, Net carb= 2g

▤ Flaxseeds (Linseeds), (1 oz (28g)): GI of 55, GL of 1, Net carb= 0g

▦ Hazelnut Butter, (2 tbsp (32g)): GI of 15, GL of 1, Net carb= 3g

▦ Hazelnuts, (1 oz (28g)): GI of 15, GL of 0, Net carb= 2g

▦ Hemp seeds, (1 oz (28g)): GI of 0, GL of 0, Net carb= 1g

▦ Macadamia Nut Butter, (2 tbsp (32g)): GI of 15, GL of 1, Net carb= 3g

▦ Macadamia nuts, (1 oz (28g)): GI of 15, GL of 1, Net carb= 2g

▦ Mustard seeds, (1 oz (28g)): GI of 15, GL of 1, Net carb= 2g

▦ Peanut Butter, (2 tbsp (32g)): GI of 13, GL of 3, Net carb= 6g

▦ Peanuts, (1 oz (28g)): GI of 13, GL of <1, Net carb= 3g

▦ Pecan Butter, (2 tbsp (32g)): GI of 0, GL of 0, Net carb= 2g

▦ Pecans, (1 oz (28g)): GI of 0, GL of 0, Net carb= 1g

▦ Pine Nut Oil, (1 tbsp (14g)): GI of 15, GL of 0, Net carb= 0g

▦ Pine nuts, (1 oz (28g)): GI of 15, GL of <1, Net carb= 4g

▦ Pistachio Butter, (2 tbsp (32g)): GI of 15, GL of <1, Net carb= 4g

▦ Pistachios, (1 oz (28g)): GI of 15, GL of <1, Net carb= 5g

▦ Poppy seeds, (1 oz (28g)): GI of 5, GL of <1, Net carb= 2g

▦ Poppy seeds, (1 oz (28g)): GI of 5, GL of <1, Net carb= 3g

▦ Pumpkin seeds (Pepitas), (1 oz (28g)): GI of 15, GL of <1, Net carb= 2g

▦ Quinoa seeds, (1 oz (28g)): GI of 53, GL of 2.2, Net carb= 4g

▦ Raw Almonds, (1 oz (28g)): GI of 0, GL of 0, Net carb= 2g

▦ Raw Brazil Nuts, (1 oz (28g)): GI of 15, GL of 0, Net carb= 1g

▦ Raw Cashews, (1 oz (28g)): GI of 25, GL of 2, Net carb= 8g

▦ Raw Chia Nuts, (1 oz (28g)): GI of 5, GL of <1, Net carb= 1g

⊞ Raw Hazelnuts (Filberts), (1 oz (28g)): GI of 15, GL of <1, Net carb= 2g

⊞ Raw Macadamia Nuts, (1 oz (28g)): GI of 15, GL of <1, Net carb= 2g

⊞ Raw Peanuts, (1 oz (28g)): GI of 13, GL of <1, Net carb= 3g

⊞ Raw Pecans, (1 oz (28g)): GI of 0, GL of 0, Net carb= 1g

⊞ Raw Pine Nuts, (1 oz (28g)): GI of 15, GL of <1, Net carb= 4g

⊞ Raw Pistachios, (1 oz (28g)): GI of 15, GL of <1, Net carb= 5g

⊞ Raw Walnuts, (1 oz (28g)): GI of 15, GL of <1, Net carb= 1g

⊞ Roasted Almonds, (1 oz (28g)): GI of 0, GL of 0, Net carb= 2g

⊞ Roasted Brazil Nuts, (1 oz (28g)): GI of 15, GL of <1, Net carb= 1g

⊞ Roasted Cashews, (1 oz (28g)): GI of 25, GL of 2, Net carb= 8g

⊞ Roasted Chestnuts, (1 oz (28g)): GI of 60, GL of 8, Net carb= 14g

⊞ Roasted Chia Nuts, (1 oz (28g)): GI of 1, GL of <1, Net carb= 1g

⊞ Roasted Hazelnuts , (1 oz (28g)): GI of 15, GL of <1, Net carb= 2g

⊞ Roasted Macadamia Nuts, (1 oz (28g)): GI of 15, GL of <1, Net carb= 2g

⊞ Roasted Peanuts, (1 oz (28g)): GI of 13, GL of <1, Net carb= 3g

⊞ Roasted Pecans, (1 oz (28g)): GI of 0, GL of 0, Net carb= 1g

⊞ Roasted Pine Nuts, (1 oz (28g)): GI of 15, GL of <1, Net carb= 4g

⊞ Roasted Pistachios, (1 oz (28g)): GI of 15, GL of <1, Net carb= 5g

⊞ Roasted Walnuts, (1 oz (28g)): GI of 15, GL of <1, Net carb= 1g

⊞ Salted Almonds, (1 oz (28g)): GI of 0, GL of 0, Net carb= 2g

⊞ Salted Brazil Nuts, (1 oz (28g)): GI of 15, GL of <1, Net carb= 1g

▤ Salted Cashews, (1 oz (28g)): GI of 25, GL of 2, Net carb= 8g

▤ Salted Hazelnuts , (1 oz (28g)): GI of 15, GL of <1, Net carb= 2g

▤ Salted Macadamia Nuts, (1 oz (28g)): GI of 15, GL of <1, Net carb= 2g

▤ Salted Peanuts, (1 oz (28g)): GI of 13, GL of <1, Net carb= 3g

▤ Salted Pecans, (1 oz (28g)): GI of 0, GL of 0, Net carb= 1g

▤ Salted Pistachios, (1 oz (28g)): GI of 15, GL of <1, Net carb= 5g

▤ Salted Walnuts, (1 oz (28g)): GI of 15, GL of <1, Net carb= 1g

▤ Sesame seeds, (1 oz (28g)): GI of 35, GL of 1, Net carb= 3g

▤ Sesame seeds, (1 oz (28g)): GI of 35, GL of 1, Net carb= 3g

▤ Steamed Chestnuts, (1 oz (28g)): GI of 60, GL of 8, Net carb= 14g

▤ Sunflower seeds, (1 oz (28g)): GI of 15, GL of <1, Net carb= 3g

▤ Tiger nuts, (1 oz (28g)): GI of 51, GL of 6, Net carb= 11g

▤ Walnut Oil, (1 tbsp (14g)): GI of 0, GL of 0, Net carb= 0g

▤ Walnuts, (1 oz (28g)): GI of 15, GL of <1, Net carb= 1g

▤ Watermelon seeds, (1 oz (28g)): GI of 10, GL of <1, Net carb= 1g

OIL AND CONDIMENTS

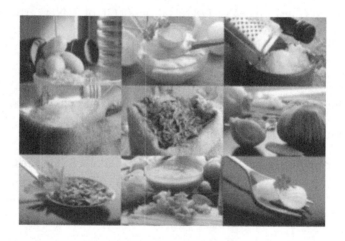

Oils, Fats, and Condiments in the DiabeteBalance Diet

Optimally managing Type 2 Diabetes (T2D) involves making informed choices about fats, oils, and condiments. These essential components not only fulfill vital bodily functions but also contribute significantly to meal enjoyment and nutritional value.

COMPLIANT OILS AND FATS:

- **Olive Oil:** Abundant in heart-healthy monounsaturated fats, olive oil can lower bad LDL cholesterol levels and enhance insulin sensitivity. Extra virgin olive oil is specifically recommended for its maximal health benefits.
- **Avocado Oil:** Rich in monounsaturated fats like olive oil, avocado oil is also suited for high-temperature cooking due to its high smoke point.
- **Canola Oil:** Balancing monounsaturated and polyunsaturated fats, canola oil is another suitable option with a high smoke point for varied cooking methods.
- **Flaxseed Oil:** Known as an excellent omega-3 source, flaxseed oil aids in reducing inflammation. Its low smoke point makes it best for cold dishes like salads.
- **Nuts and Seeds:** Almonds, walnuts, flaxseeds, chia seeds, sunflower seeds, and hemp seeds are all nutritious choices, rich in beneficial fats, fiber, and protein.
- **Fatty Fish:** Salmon, mackerel, sardines, and trout provide essential omega-3 fatty acids for heart health and inflammation control.
- **Coconut Oil:** Though higher in saturated fats, coconut oil can still be used in moderation for its unique flavor and medium-chain fatty acids.

Cooking Methods:

Grilling, roasting, steaming, sautéing, and baking are preferable to deep frying to avoid harmful compound formation.

COMPLIANT CONDIMENTS:

- **Mustard:** Dijon or whole-grain mustards are low-sugar, low-calorie choices.
- **Vinegar:** Apple cider, balsamic, white and red wine vinegars offer flavorful options without causing significant spikes in blood sugar levels.
- **Salsa:** Homemade salsa from fresh ingredients provides a nutrient-rich, low-calorie option.
- **Herbs and Spices:** Rosemary, thyme, oregano, garlic, turmeric, cinnamon, and more add flavor without extra calories or sugars.
- **Homemade Dressings:** Combining compliant oils with vinegar, herbs, and spices lets you avoid added sugars and unhealthy fats.
- **Sugar-free or Low-sodium Sauces:** Store-bought options aligned with the DiabeteBalance Diet can also be suitable if chosen carefully.
- **Greek Yogurt:** Used as a base for creamy dressings, Greek yogurt adds protein without excessive fat or sugar.

HERBS AND SPICES

Herbs and spices form a fundamental aspect of any diet aimed at optimally managing diabetes. They contribute unique flavors, complexity, and numerous health benefits to meals. Understanding their role in controlling glycemic load and aligning with the DiabeteBalance Diet is crucial. Let's delve into the potential benefits, drawbacks, and practical ways to incorporate them into the diet.

Benefits of Herbs and Spices:

- **Antioxidant-rich:** Oregano, cinnamon, turmeric, and others are packed with antioxidants, combating oxidative stress, a condition linked to chronic diseases like T2D.
- **Blood Sugar Regulation:** Some, such as cinnamon and fenugreek seeds, can lessen insulin resistance and decrease fasting blood glucose levels, enhancing insulin sensitivity.
- **Anti-Inflammatory:** Herbs and spices like garlic, curcuma, cardamom, turmeric and ginger possess potent anti-inflammatory properties, beneficial for conditions like T2D, where chronic inflammation is often present.

Drawbacks of Herbs and Spices:

- **Interactions with Medications:** Certain ones may interfere with diabetes medications. Cinnamon, for example, could cause blood sugar to drop too low. Consult with healthcare professionals to avoid adverse interactions.
- **Quality and Purity:** Not all are equal in quality. Some might contain additives or contaminants, emphasizing the need for purchasing high-quality products from reliable sources.
- **Overconsumption:** Though beneficial, excessive intake may cause digestive issues or other side effects, underscoring the importance of moderation.

Incorporating Herbs and Spices into the DiabeteBalance Diet:

- **Diversify Your Selection:** Explore various herbs and spices to enjoy a broad range of antioxidants and healthful compounds.
- **Use in Cooking:** Substitute unhealthy ingredients like salt or sugar with herbs and spices, adding flavor without extra calories or sodium.
- **Consult a Professional:** For guidance on specific health benefits or if considering larger-than-usual amounts, consult your healthcare provider.
- **Consider Fresh and Dried:** Both forms offer benefits, allowing you to choose based on availability and cooking needs.
- **Tea Infusions:** Experiment with tea infusions like ginger or cinnamon tea for a comforting beverage that supports blood sugar management.

Comprehensive Food Selection:

Herbs and spices add richness to the culinary experience, and their therapeutic properties can be harnessed in the fight against T2D. By integrating them responsibly and creatively, they can be powerful allies in aligning with the DiabeteBalance Diet, enhancing both flavor and health.

The following list provides a comprehensive selection of foods that fully comply with the DiabeteBalance Diet. Information on serving size, Glycemic Index (GI), Glycemic Load (GL), and Net Carbohydrates equips you to make informed decisions for portion sizes and effective meal planning. The foods are sorted alphabetically for easy reference.

▤ Allspice, (1 tsp (2.1 g)): GI of 15 (Low), GL of 0.3 (Low)

▤ Anise seeds, (1 tsp (2.1 g)): GI of 0.0 (Low), GL of 0.3 (Low)

▤ Asian chives, (1 tbsp (3 g)): GI of 15 (Low), GL of 0.3 (Low)

▤ Basil, (1 tsp (0.7 g)): GI of 70 (High), GL of 0 (Low)

▤ Bay leaves, (1 tbsp, crumbled (1.8 g)): GI of 23 (Low), GL of 0.1 (Low)

▤ Black cumin, (1 tsp (2.4 g)): GI of 0.0 (Low), GL of 0.3 (Low)

▤ Black pepper, (1 tsp (2.4 g)): GI of 44 (Low), GL of 0.3 (Low)

▤ capers, (1 tbsp (8.6 g)): GI of 20 (Low), GL of 1.4 (Low)

▤ Caraway, (1 tbsp (6.7 g)): GI of 5 (Low), GL of 1.1 (Low)

▤ Cardamom, (1 tbsp (5.8 g)): GI of 82 (High), GL of 1 (Low)

▤ Celery seed, (1 tbsp (5.8 g)): GI of 32 (Low), GL of 0.9 (Low)

▤ Chiles, (1 tbsp (8 g)): GI of 42 (Low), GL of 1.3 (Low)

▤ chilli, (1 tbsp (8 g)): GI of 15 (Low), GL of 1.3 (Low)

▤ Chives, (1 tbsp (2.8 g)): GI of 15 (Low), GL of 0.3 (Low)

▤ Cinnamon, (1 tbsp (7.9 g)): GI of 70 (High), GL of 2.1 (Low)

▦ Cloves, (1 tbsp (6.6 g)): GI of 87 (High), GL of 3.5 (Low)

▦ Coriander seed, (1 tbsp (5 g)): GI of 33 (Low), GL of 1 (Low)

▦ Cumin, (1 tbsp (6 g)): GI of 0.0 (Low), GL of 0 (Low)

▦ Curry Leaves, (5 leaves (2g)): GI of 5 (Low), GL of 0.1 (Low)

▦ Curry powder, (1 tbsp (6 g)): GI of 5 (Low), GL of 0.4 (Low)

▦ Dill seed, (1 tsp (2.4 g)): GI of 15 (Low), GL of 0.3 (Low)

▦ Fennel seeds, (1 tbsp (5.8 g)): GI of 16 (Low), GL of 0.3 (Low)

▦ Fenugreek Leaves, (1 cup (85 g)): GI of 25 (Low), GL of 0.6 (Low)

▦ Fenugreek, (1 tbsp (11.1 g)): GI of 25 (Low), GL of 0.6 (Low)

▦ Five Spice Powder, (1 tsp (2.1 g)): GI of 15 (Low), GL of 0.4 (Low)

▦ Garlic chives, (2 clove (6 g)): GI of 15 (Low), GL of 1 (Low)

▦ Ginger, (1 tsp (2.1 g)): GI of 72 (High), GL of 0.3 (Low)

▦ Lemon Balm, (1 tsp (2.1 g)): GI of 15 (Low), GL of 0.3 (Low)

▦ Lemongrass, (1 cup (67 g)): GI of 45 (Low), GL of 7.4 (Low)

▦ Lime Leaves, (5 leaves (2 g)): GI of 32 (Low), GL of 0.4 (Low)

▦ Mint, (1 tbsp (3.1 g)): GI of 10 (Low), GL of 0.2 (Low)

▦ Mustard Seed, (1 tsp (2 g)): GI of 32 (Low), GL of 0.2 (Low)

▦ Nutmeg, (1 tsp (2.4 g)): GI of 46 (Low), GL of 0.3 (Low)

▦ Oregano, (1 tbsp (3 g)): GI of 5 (Low), GL of 0.3 (Low)

▦ Paprika, (1 tsp (2 g)): GI of 15 (Low), GL of 0.3 (Low)

▦ Poppy seeds, (1 tbsp (8.8 g)): GI of 5 (Low), GL of 0.1 (Low)

▦ Rosemary, (1 tbsp (3.3 g)): GI of 70 (High), GL of 1.1 (Low)

▦ Saffron, (1 tsp (0.7 g)): GI of 70 (High), GL of 0.2 (Low)

■ Sage, (1 tsp (0.7 g)): GI of 15 (Low), GL of 0.2 (Low)

■ Savory, (1 tbsp (4.4 g)): GI of 16 (Low), GL of 0.2 (Low)

■ Sesame seeds, (1 tbsp (10 g)): GI of 31 (Low), GL of 0.1 (Low)

■ Sumac, (1 tsp (2.7 g)): GI of 43 (Low), GL of 0.2 (Low)

■ Summer Savoy, (1 tsp (2.7 g)): GI of 21 (Low), GL of 0.2 (Low)

■ Tarragon, (1 tbsp (1.8g)): GI of 15 (Low), GL of 0.1 (Low)

■ Thyme, (1 tbsp, leaves (2.7 g)): GI of 51 (Low), GL of 0.1 (Low)

■ Turmeric, (1 tbsp (6.8 g)): GI of 15 (Low), GL of 0.5 (Low)

■ Vanilla, (1 tbsp (4.4 g)): GI of 16 (Low), GL of 0.5 (Low)

■ Wasabi powder, (1 tsp (2.8 g)): GI of 31 (Low), GL of 0.3 (Low)

■ Watercress, (1 cup, chopped (34 g)): GI of 32 (Low), GL of 0.1 (Low)

■ Wild garlic, (1 oz (28 g)): GI of 11 (Low), GL of 2 (Low)

VEGETABLES AND VEGETABLE PRODUCTS

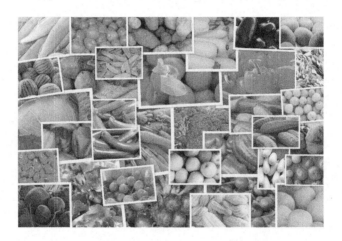

Vegetables and vegetable products are foundational pillars in various diets around the world, reflecting the diversity and richness of cultures and cuisines. Their array of colors, textures, and flavors, contribute not only to the culinary palette but also to nutritional well-being. In the context of a balanced diet, vegetables serve as rich sources of essential vitamins, minerals, and fiber, playing a vital role in promoting digestive health, reducing the likelihood of chronic diseases, and supporting immune function. Particularly for those following specialized diets, like the DiabeteBalance Diet, understanding the glycemic load and nutrient content of different vegetables can be crucial. While raw vegetables often retain maximum nutrients, even processed or cooked vegetable products can offer health benefits when chosen wisely. By integrating a diverse range of vegetables and their products into one's diet, individuals can achieve a harmonious blend of taste and health, supporting not only diabetes management but overall vitality.

Benefits of Vegetables and Vegetable Products:

- **Nutrient-Dense:** They supply essential nutrients such as vitamins, minerals, fiber, and antioxidants, boosting overall health.
- **Low in Calories:** Most vegetables are low-calorie, supporting weight management.
- **High in Fiber:** The fiber content helps slow sugar absorption, preventing sudden spikes in blood glucose and insulin.

Considerations on Juices, Sodium, and Cooking Methods:

Fruit and Vegetable Juices: Although nutrient-rich, juices often lack fiber and are high in sugar. Opt for whole fruits and vegetables instead.

High Sodium Preparations: Some canned or pre-packaged products contain excessive sodium. Check labels for low-sodium or no-salt-added options.

Cooking Methods: Avoid methods that add fats or lose nutrients, such as deep frying or boiling. Opt for steaming, sautéing, grilling, roasting, or eating raw to preserve nutritional value.

Potential Drawbacks:

- **Starchy Vegetables:** Potatoes, corn, and peas, among others, can raise blood glucose if not moderated.

- **Processed Products:** Canned vegetables or juices with added sugars, sodium, or additives can be less suitable for diabetes management.

Incorporating Vegetables into the DiabeteBalance Diet:

- **Emphasize Non-Starchy Vegetables:** Focus on low-carb options like leafy greens, broccoli, bell peppers, and zucchini.
- **Monitor Portion Sizes:** Be mindful of portions, especially for starchy vegetables with higher carbohydrate content.
- **Choose Fresh or Frozen Over Canned:** Avoid added sodium by selecting fresh or frozen produce.
- **Read Labels Diligently:** Look for minimal added sugars, sodium, or other additives when shopping.

Comprehensive Food Selection:

Vegetables and vegetable products are invaluable in DiabeteBalance diet. By understanding their benefits and being mindful of potential pitfalls, you can make informed choices that promote both diabetes management and overall wellness. The Diet emphasizes whole, unprocessed foods, minimal sugars, and healthy preparation methods, making it an excellent framework for incorporating these nutritious foods into your daily regimen.

The following list offers foods that align with the DiabeteBalance Diet, detailing serving size, Glycemic Index (GI), Glycemic Load (GL), and Net Carbohydrates. This equips you with the tools for intelligent portion control and meal planning.

LOW GLYCEMIC LOAD FOODS A-Z

Alfalfa Sprouts, (1 cup (33g)): GI of 15, GL of 1, Net carb= 0.4g

▤ Amaranth Leaves Cooked Boiled With Salt Drained, (1 cup (132g)): GI of 65, GL of 4, Net carb= 5.4g

▤ Amaranth Leaves Cooked Boiled Without Salt Drained, (1 cup (132g)): GI of 65, GL of 4, Net carb= 5.4g

▤ Artichoke Dip, (2 tbsp (30g)): GI of 15, GL of 1, Net carb= 2g

▤ Artichoke Hearts, (1 cup (168g)): GI of 20, GL of 5, Net carb= 12g

▤ Artichoke, (1 medium (120g)): GI of 20, GL of 3, Net carb= 9g

▤ Artichokes, (globe or french), raw, (1 medium (120g)): GI of 15-20, GL of 4, Net carb= 4.2g

▤ Arugula, raw, (1 cup (20g)): GI of 20-30, GL of 0, Net carb= 0.4g

▤ Asparagus Chips, (1 oz (28g)): GI of 15, GL of 1, Net carb= 7g

▤ Asparagus Pea, (1 cup (90g)): GI of 15-20, GL of 1, Net carb= 4g

▤ Asparagus Puree, (1/2 cup (125g)): GI of 15, GL of 1, Net carb= 4g

▤ Asparagus, (1 cup (134g)): GI of 15, GL of 1, Net carb= 4g

▤ Avocado, (1/2 avocado (100g)): GI of 15, GL of 0, Net carb= 2g

▤ Baba Ghanoush, (2 tbsp (30g)): GI of 15, GL of 1, Net carb= 3g

▤ Balsam-pear (bitter gourd), leafy tips, raw, (1 cup (64g)): GI of 15-25, GL of 1, Net carb= 1.6g

▤ Balsam-pear (bitter gourd), pods, raw, (1 cup (93g)): GI of 15-25, GL of 1, Net carb= 2.3g

▤ Bamboo Shoots, (1 cup (151g)): GI of 15, GL of 1, Net carb= 3g

▤ Bean Sprouts, (1 cup (104g)): GI of 30, GL of 2, Net carb= 4g

▤ Beans, fava, in pod, raw, (1 cup (130g)): GI of 20-30, GL of 2, Net carb= 7.8g

▤ Beans, kidney, mature seeds, soaked and cooked, (1 cup (104g)): GI of 25-40, GL of 3, Net carb= 3.7g

▤ Beans, navy, mature seeds, soaked and cooked, (1 cup (104g)): GI of 20-30, GL of 1, Net carb= 2.8g

▤ Beans, pinto, mature seeds, soaked and cooked, (1 cup (104g)): GI of 25-40, GL of 2, Net carb= 5.5g

▤ Beans, snap, green, soaked and cooked, (1 cup (100g)): GI of 45219, GL of 1, Net carb= 3.9g

▤ Beans, snap, yellow, , soaked and cooked, (1 cup (100g)): GI of 20-30, GL of 1, Net carb= 3.2g

▤ Beet Chips, (1 oz (28g)): GI of 61, GL of 5, Net carb= 11g

▤ Beet Greens, Cooked with salt, (1 cup (144g)): GI of 15, GL of 1, Net carb= 3g

▤ Beet Greens, Cooked without salt, (1 cup (144g)): GI of 15, GL of 1, Net carb= 3g

▤ Beet Greens, Raw, (1 cup (144g)): GI of 15, GL of 1, Net carb= 3g

▤ Beetroot Powder, (1 tbsp (8g)): GI of 61, GL of 2, Net carb= 5g

▤ Beetroot Puree, (1/2 cup (125g)): GI of 61, GL of 7, Net carb= 14g

▤ Beets Cooked Boiled. Drained With Salt, (1 cup (136g)): GI of 60-70, GL of 5, Net carb= 13g

▤ Beets, cooked without salt, (1 cup (136g)): GI of 64, GL of 7, Net carb= 13g

▤ Beets, raw, (1 cup (136g)): GI of 60-70, GL of 5, Net carb= 13g

▤ Bell Peppers, (1 cup (149g)): GI of 15, GL of 1, Net carb= 6g

▤ Bitter Melon, Cooked with salt, (1/2 cup (100g)): GI of 15-30, GL of 3, Net carb= 4g

▤ Bitter Melon, (1/2 cup (100g)): GI of 15-30, GL of 3, Net carb= 4g

▤ Black Beans, (1 cup (172g)): GI of 30, GL of 8, Net carb= 24g

▤ Bok Choy, Cooked, (1 cup (170g)): GI of 15, GL of 0, Net carb= 1g

▤ Bok Choy, Raw, (1 cup (170g)): GI of 15, GL of 0, Net carb= 1g

▤ Borage Cooked Boiled Drained With Salt, (1 cup (89g)): GI of 15-20, GL of 1, Net carb= 0.6g

▤ Borage Cooked Boiled Drained Without Salt, (1 cup (89g)): GI of 15-20, GL of 1, Net carb= 0.6g

▤ Borage, raw, (1 cup (89g)): GI of 15-20, GL of 1, Net carb= 0.6g

▤ Broccoflower Cooked, (1 cup (100g)): GI of 15, GL of 1, Net carb= 3g

▤ Broccoflower, Raw, (1 cup (100g)): GI of 15, GL of 1, Net carb= 3g

▤ Broccoli Powder, (1 tbsp (7g)): GI of 15, GL of 1, Net carb= 4.4g

▤ Broccoli Puree, (1/2 cup (125g)): GI of 15, GL of 1, Net carb= 6g

▤ Broccoli raab, raw, (1 cup (40g)): GI of 15-20, GL of 1, Net carb= 0.7g

▤ Broccoli Stem Noodles, (1 cup (100g)): GI of 15, GL of 1, Net carb= 3g

▤ Broccoli, Chinese, raw, (1 cup (56g)): GI of 15-20, GL of 1, Net carb= 1.8g

▤ Broccoli, leaves, raw, (1 cup (50g)): GI of 15-20, GL of 1, Net carb= 1.4g

▤ Broccoli, (1 cup (156g)): GI of 15, GL of 1, Net carb= 6g

▤ Broccoli, stalks, raw, (1 cup (92g)): GI of 15-20, GL of 1, Net carb= 3.3g

▤ Brussels Sprouts Chips, (1 oz (28g)): GI of 15, GL of 1, Net carb= 7g

▤ Brussels Sprouts, Cooked, (1 cup (156g)): GI of 15, GL of 2, Net carb= 8g

▤ Burdock root, Cooked without salt, (1 cup (116g)): GI of 40-50, GL of 7, Net carb= 14.3g

▤ Burdock root, raw, (1 cup (116g)): GI of 40-50, GL of 7, Net carb= 14.3g

▤ Burdock, Cooked, Boiled with salt, (1 cup (116g)): GI of 40-50, GL of 7, Net carb= 14.3g

▤ Butterbur (fuki), raw, (1 cup (55g)): GI of 15-20, GL of 1, Net carb= 1.5g

▤ Butternut Squash Noodles, (1 cup (150g)): GI of 51, GL of 5, Net carb= 13g

▤ Butternut Squash Puree, (1/2 cup (125g)): GI of 51, GL of 7, Net carb= 14g

▤ Butternut Squash, (1 cup (205g)): GI of 51, GL of 8, Net carb= 21g

▤ Cabbage Green, Cooked without salt, (1 cup (205g)): GI of 15, GL of 1, Net carb= 4g

▤ Cabbage, chinese (pak-choi), raw, (1 cup (70g)): GI of 15-20, GL of 1, Net carb= 1g

▤ Cabbage, chinese (pe-tsai), cooked without salt, (1 cup (76g)): GI of 15-20, GL of 1, Net carb= 1.2g

▤ Cabbage, chinese (pe-tsai), raw, (1 cup (76g)): GI of 15-20, GL of 1, Net carb= 1.2g

▤ Cabbage, raw, (1 cup (89g)): GI of 15-20, GL of 1, Net carb= 3g

▤ Cabbage, red, raw, (1 cup (89g)): GI of 15-20, GL of 1, Net carb= 4g

▤ Cabbage, savoy, raw, (1 cup (70g)): GI of 15-20, GL of 1, Net carb= 2.5g

▤ Canned Acorn Squash, (1 cup (245g)): GI of 15, GL of 1, Net carb= 7g

▤ Canned Artichoke Hearts, (1 cup (168g)): GI of 15, GL of 2, Net carb= 8g

▤ Canned Asparagus, (1 cup (200g)): GI of 15, GL of 1, Net carb= 6g

▤ Canned Bamboo Shoots, (1 cup (151g)): GI of 15, GL of 1, Net carb= 5g

▤ Canned butternut Squash, (1 cup (245g)): GI of 15, GL of 1, Net carb= 7g

▤ Canned Carrots, (1 cup (236g)): GI of 39, GL of 7, Net carb= 18g

▤ Canned Green Beans, (1 cup (240g)): GI of 15, GL of 3, Net carb= 12g

▤ Canned Lima Beans, (1 cup (240g)): GI of 20, GL of 5, Net carb= 12g

▤ Canned Mixed Vegetables, (1 cup (240g)): GI of 45, GL of 7, Net carb= 16g

▤ Canned Mushrooms, (1 cup (156g)): GI of 15, GL of 1, Net carb= 4g

▤ Canned Okra, (1 cup (256g)): GI of 15, GL of 1, Net carb= 4g

▤ Canned Olives, (1 ounce (28g)): GI of 15, GL of 0, Net carb= 1g

▤ Canned Pickles, (1 spear (35g)): GI of 15, GL of 0, Net carb= 1g

▤ Canned Pumpkin, (1 cup (245g)): GI of 15, GL of 3, Net carb= 12g

▤ Canned Sauerkraut, (1 cup (142g)): GI of 15, GL of 1, Net carb= 4g

▤ Canned Spaghetti Squash, (1 cup (245g)): GI of 15, GL of 1, Net carb= 7g

▤ Canned Spinach, (1 cup (214g)): GI of 15, GL of 1, Net carb= 4g

▤ Canned Tomatoes, (1 cup (240g)): GI of 45, GL of 6, Net carb= 13g

▤ Canned Water Chestnuts, (1 cup (140g)): GI of 54, GL of 7, Net carb= 14g

▤ Cardoon Cooked Boiled with salt and drained, (1 cup (150g)): GI of 15-20, GL of 1, Net carb= 3.5g

▤ Cardoon Cooked Boiled with salt and drained, (1 cup (150g)): GI of 15-20, GL of 1, Net carb= 3.5g

▤ Cardoon, raw, (1 cup (120g)): GI of 15-20, GL of 1, Net carb= 3.5g

▤ Carrot Chips, (1 oz (28g)): GI of 47, GL of 4, Net carb= 9g

▤ Carrot Greens, (1 cup (25g)): GI of 15, GL of 0, Net carb= 1g

▤ Carrot Noodles, (1 cup (110g)): GI of 47, GL of 4, Net carb= 8g

▤ Carrot Powder, (1 tbsp (7g)): GI of 47, GL of 1, Net carb= 3g

▤ Carrot Puree, (1/2 cup (125g)): GI of 47, GL of 7, Net carb= 14g

▤ Carrot Spread, (2 tbsp (30g)): GI of 35, GL of 2, Net carb= 4g

▤ Carrots, baby, raw, (1 cup (128g)): GI of 45-55, GL of 6, Net carb= 11.5g

▤ Cauliflower Cooked With Salt, Boiled and Drained, (1 cup (56g)): GI of 15, GL of 1, Net carb= 2g

▤ Cauliflower Frozen Unprepared, (1 cup (56g)): GI of 15, GL of 1, Net carb= 2g

▤ Cauliflower Green Cooked With Salt, (1 cup (56g)): GI of 15, GL of 1, Net carb= 2g

▤ Cauliflower Greens, (1 cup (56g)): GI of 15, GL of 1, Net carb= 2g

▤ Cauliflower Powder, (1 tbsp (6g)): GI of 15, GL of 0, Net carb= 1g

▤ Cauliflower Puree, (1/2 cup (125g)): GI of 15, GL of 1, Net carb= 4g

▤ Celeriac Cooked Boiled With Salt Drained, (1/2 cup (125g)): GI of 15, GL of 1, Net carb= 6g

▤ Celeriac Cooked without salt, (1 cup (156g)): GI of 15, GL of 2, Net carb= 9g

▤ Celeriac Puree, (1/2 cup (125g)): GI of 15, GL of 1, Net carb= 6g

▤ Celeriac, (1 cup (156g)): GI of 15, GL of 1, Net carb= 6g

▤ Celery Powder, (1 tbsp (6g)): GI of 15, GL of 0, Net carb= 1g

▤ Celery Root Puree, (1/2 cup (125g)): GI of 15, GL of 1, Net carb= 6g

▤ Celery, (1 cup (101g)): GI of 15, GL of 0, Net carb= 2g

▤ Chard Cooked, (1 cup (175g)): GI of 15, GL of 1, Net carb= 5g

▤ Chayote Cooked Boiled with salt Drained, (1 cup (132g)): GI of 15, GL of 1, Net carb= 4g

▤ Chayote Fruit Raw, (1 cup (132g)): GI of 15, GL of 1, Net carb= 4g

▤ Chickpeas, (½ cup (82g)): GI of 28, GL of 4, Net carb= 13.5g

▤ Chicory greens, raw, (1 cup (55g)): GI of 15-20, GL of 1, Net carb= 0.5g

▤ Chicory roots, raw, (1 cup (60g)): GI of 20-25, GL of 1, Net carb= 4g

▤ Chicory, witloof, raw, (1 cup (50g)): GI of 15-20, GL of 1, Net carb= 0.8g

▤ Chives, (1 tbsp (3g)): GI of 15, GL of 0, Net carb= 0g

▤ Chrysanthemum leaves, raw, (1 cup (43g)): GI of 15-20, GL of 1, Net carb= 0.6g

▤ Chrysanthemum, garland, Cooked Boiled With Salt Drained, (1 cup (20g)): GI of 15-20, GL of 1, Net carb= 1.2g

▤ Collard Greens, Cooked , (1 cup (190g)): GI of 15, GL of 1, Net carb= 5g

▤ Collards Chopped Unprepared, (1 cup (190g)): GI of 15, GL of 1, Net carb= 5g

▤ Cornsalad, raw, (1 cup (56g)): GI of 15-20, GL of 1, Net carb= 1.5g

▤ Cowpeas, leafy tips, raw, (1 cup (36g)): GI of 15-20, GL of 1, Net carb= 1g

▤ Cowpeas, young pods with seeds, raw, (1 cup (100g)): GI of 35-40, GL of 4, Net carb= 8g

▤ Cress Garden Cooked Boiled With Salt Drained, (1 cup (25g)): GI of 15-20, GL of 1, Net carb= 0.7g

▤ Cress, garden, raw, (1 cup (25g)): GI of 15-20, GL of 1, Net carb= 0.7g

▤ Cucumber Chips, (1 oz (28g)): GI of 15, GL of 1, Net carb= 6g

▤ Cucumber Noodles, (1 cup (100g)): GI of 15, GL of 0, Net carb= 2g

▤ Cucumber, peeled, raw, (1 cup (133g)): GI of 15, GL of 1, Net carb= 2.5g

▤ Cucumber, (1 cup (104g)): GI of 15, GL of 0, Net carb= 2g

▤ Cucumber, with peel, raw, (1 cup (104g)): GI of 15, GL of 1, Net carb= 3g

▤ Daikon Radish Noodles, (1 cup (120g)): GI of 15, GL of 1, Net carb= 3g

▤ Daikon, (1 cup (116g)): GI of 15, GL of 1, Net carb= 4g

▤ Dandelion Greens Cooked Boiled With Salt Drained, (1 cup (55g)): GI of 15, GL of 1, Net carb= 3g

▤ Dandelion Greens, Cooked without salt, (1 cup (55g)): GI of 15, GL of 1, Net carb= 3g

▤ Dandelion Greens, Raw, (1 cup (55g)): GI of 15, GL of 1, Net carb= 3g

▤ Dock, raw, (1 cup (133g)): GI of 15-20, GL of 1, Net carb= 2g

▤ Drumstick Leaves Cooked Boiled Drained With Salt, (1/2 cup (100g)): GI of 15-20, GL of 1, Net carb= 0.5g

▦ Drumstick leaves, raw, (1 cup (21g)): GI of 15-20, GL of 1, Net carb= 0.5g

▦ Drumstick pods, raw, (1 cup (99g)): GI of 20-25, GL of 2, Net carb= 4g

▦ Edamame Cooked, (1 cup (155g)): GI of 15, GL of 3, Net carb= 8g

▦ Edamame Unprepared, (1/2 cup (75g)): GI of 15, GL of 3, Net carb= 8g

▦ Eggplant Noodles, (1 cup (100g)): GI of 15, GL of 0, Net carb= 2g

▦ Eggplant, Raw, (1 cup (99g)): GI of 15, GL of 1, Net carb= 6g

▦ Endive Leaves, (1 cup (40g)): GI of 15, GL of 0, Net carb= 1g

▦ Endive, (1 cup (50g)): GI of 15, GL of 0, Net carb= 1g

▦ Epazote, raw, (1 cup (20g)): GI of 15-20, GL of 1, Net carb= 0.7g

▦ Eppaw, raw, (1 cup (20g)): GI of 15-20, GL of 1, Net carb= 1g

▦ Escarole Cooked without salt, (1 cup (75g)): GI of 15, GL of 1, Net carb= 3g

▦ Escarole Creamed, (1 cup (75g)): GI of 15, GL of 1, Net carb= 3g

▦ Fennel Bulb Cooked Boiled with salt drained, (1 cup (87g)): GI of 15, GL of 1, Net carb= 5g

▦ Fennel Puree, (½ cup (125g)): GI of 15, GL of 1, Net carb= 5g

▦ Fennel Sliced Serving size 1 cup (87g): GI of 15, (1 cup (87g)): GI of 15, GL of 1, Net carb= 4g

▦ Fiddlehead ferns, raw, (1 cup (87g)): GI of 15-20, GL of 1, Net carb= 4g

▦ Fireweed, leaves, raw, (1 cup (35g)): GI of 15-20, GL of 1, Net carb= 1.5g

▦ Garlic Powder, (1 teaspoon (3g)): GI of 15, GL of 0, Net carb= 1g

Garlic Scapes, (1 cup (40g)): GI of 15, GL of 0, Net carb= 1g

Garlic, (1 clove (3g)): GI of 15, GL of 0, Net carb= 1g

Ginger root, raw, (1 tbsp (9g)): GI of 15-20, GL of 1, Net carb= 1g

Ginger, (1 tbsp (6g)): GI of 15, GL of 0, Net carb= 1g

Gourd, dishcloth (towelgourd), raw, (1 cup (86g)): GI of 15-20, GL of 1, Net carb= 2g

Gourd, white-flowered (calabash), raw, (1 cup (116g)): GI of 15-20, GL of 1, Net carb= 3g

Grape Leaves Canned, (1 cup (28g)): GI of 15-20, GL of 1, Net carb= 1.5g

Grape leaves, raw, (1 cup (28g)): GI of 15-20, GL of 1, Net carb= 1.5g

Green Bean Chips, (1 oz (28g)): GI of 15, GL of 1, Net carb= 6g

Green Beans, (1 cup (125g)): GI of 15, GL of 1, Net carb= 5g

Green Bell Pepper Powder, (1 tbsp (6g)): GI of 15, GL of 0, Net carb= 2g

Green Onion, (1 cup (100g)): GI of 15, GL of 1, Net carb= 4g

Guacamole, (2 tbsp (30g)): GI of 15, GL of 1, Net carb= 2g

Hearts of palm, raw, (1 cup (146g)): GI of 15-20, GL of 1, Net carb= 4g

Hubbard Squash, (1 cup (205g)): GI of 50, GL of 6, Net carb= 16g

Hummus, (2 tbsp (30g)): GI of 25, GL of 2, Net carb= 4g

Jalapeno, (1 pepper (14g)): GI of 15, GL of 0, Net carb= 1g

Jerusalem Artichoke, Cooked , (½ cup (75g)): GI of 50, GL of 3, Net carb= 11g

▤ Jerusalem Artichokes Raw, (½ cup (150g)): GI of 50, GL of 3, Net carb= 11g

▤ Jicama Chips, (1 oz (28g)): GI of 15, GL of 1, Net carb= 6g

▤ Jicama Noodles, (1 cup (120g)): GI of 15, GL of 2, Net carb= 5g

▤ Jicama, (1 cup (120g)): GI of 15, GL of 2, Net carb= 6g

▤ Jute, potherb, raw, (1 cup (28g)): GI of 15-20, GL of 1, Net carb= 0.5g

▤ Kale Chips, (1 oz (28g)): GI of 15, GL of 1, Net carb= 6g

▤ Kale Cooked Boiled With Salt Drained, (1 cup (130g)): GI of 15, GL of 1, Net carb= 4g

▤ Kale Cooked Boiled Without Salt Drained, (1 cup (130g)): GI of 15, GL of 1, Net carb= 4g

▤ Kale Powder, (1 tbsp (6g)): GI of 15, GL of 0, Net carb= 1g

▤ Kale, (1 cup (130g)): GI of 15, GL of 1, Net carb= 4g

▤ Kelp, (1 cup (76g)): GI of 15, GL of 0, Net carb= 1g

▤ Kohlrabi Noodles, (1 cup (135g)): GI of 15, GL of 1, Net carb= 5g

▤ Kohlrabi, (1 cup (135g)): GI of 15, GL of 2, Net carb= 8g

▤ Lambsquarters, raw, (1 cup (28g)): GI of 15-20, GL of 1, Net carb= 1g

▤ Leek Leaves, (1 cup (72g)): GI of 15, GL of 1, Net carb= 4g

▤ Lemon grass (citronella), raw, (1 tbsp (6g)): GI of 15-20, GL of 1, Net carb= 0.4g

▤ Lemon Juice with Cayenne Pepper and Turmeric, (1 cup (240ml)): GI of 22, GL of 2, Net carb= 6g

▤ Lentils Sprouted Cooked Stir-Fried With Salt, (1 cup (198g)): GI of 29, GL of 7, Net carb= 27g

▤ Lentils Sprouts, (½ cup (98g)): GI of 29, GL of 3.5, Net carb= 13.5g

▤ Lettuce, green leaf, raw, (1 cup (36g)): GI of 15, GL of 1, Net carb= 1g

▤ Lettuce, iceberg (includes crisphead types), raw, (1 cup (72g)): GI of 15, GL of 1, Net carb= 1g

▤ Lettuce, red leaf, raw, (1 cup (28g)): GI of 15, GL of 1, Net carb= 0.7g

▤ Lettuce, Romaine, (1 cup (72g)): GI of 15, GL of 0, Net carb= 1g

▤ Lotus Root, (1 cup (120g)): GI of 60, GL of 7, Net carb= 16g

▤ Mung Bean Sprouts, (1 cup (104g)): GI of 30, GL of 2, Net carb= 4g

▤ Mung Beans Mature Seeds Sprouted Cooked Stir-Fried, (1 cup (104g)): GI of 30, GL of 2, Net carb= 4g

▤ Mung Beans, Sprouted Cooked Boiled With Salt Drained, (1 cup (104g)): GI of 30, GL of 2, Net carb= 4g

▤ Mung Beans, Sprouted Cooked Boiled Without Salt Drained, (1 cup (104g)): GI of 30, GL of 2, Net carb= 4g

▤ Mushroom Powder, (1 tbsp (7g)): GI of 15, GL of 0, Net carb= 1g

▤ Mushroom, (1 cup (70g)): GI of 15, GL of 0, Net carb= 2g

▤ Mushrooms (Portobello, Shiitake, etc.), (1 cup (86g)): GI of 15, GL of 0, Net carb= 2g

▤ Mustard Spinach (Tendergreen) Cooked Boiled With Salt Drained, (1 cup (140g)): GI of 15-20, GL of 1, Net carb= 1.5g

▤ Mustard spinach (tendergreen), raw, (1 cup (56g)): GI of 15-20, GL of 1, Net carb= 1.5g

▤ Napa Cabbage, (1 cup (109g)): GI of 15, GL of 1, Net carb= 3g

▤ New Zealand spinach, raw, (1 cup (56g)): GI of 15-20, GL of 1, Net carb= 1g

▦ Nopales, (1 cup (86g)): GI of 15, GL of 1, Net carb= 3g

▦ Okra, (1 cup (100g)): GI of 15, GL of 1, Net carb= 4g

▦ Olives, Black, (1 ounce (28g)): GI of 15, GL of 0, Net carb= 1g

▦ Olives, Green, (1 ounce (28g)): GI of 15, GL of 0, Net carb= 1g

▦ Onion Cooked, (1 cup (160g)): GI of 15, GL of 4, Net carb= 15g

▦ Onion Juice, (1 tbsp (15ml)): GI of 15, GL of 0, Net carb= 1g

▦ Onion Powder, (1 teaspoon (2g)): GI of 15, GL of 0, Net carb= 1g

▦ Onions Welsh Raw, (1 cup (160g)): GI of 15, GL of 4, Net carb= 15g

▦ Onions, spring or scallions, raw, (1 cup (100g)): GI of 30-35, GL of 3, Net carb= 6g

▦ Onions, sweet, raw, (1 cup (160g)): GI of 30-35, GL of 5, Net carb= 14g

▦ Onions, welsh, raw, (1 cup (100g)): GI of 30-35, GL of 3, Net carb= 7g

▦ Parsnip, (½ cup (78g)): GI of 52, GL of 6, Net carb= 12g

▦ Parsley (10%) and Lemon (60%) Juice, (1 cup (240ml)): GI of 15, GL of 1, Net carb= 7g

▦ Parsley Juice 30%, (1 cup (240ml)): GI of 15, GL of 1, Net carb= 6g

▦ Parsley, (1 tbsp (3g)): GI of 15, GL of 0, Net carb= 0g

▦ Parsnip Puree, (½ cup (125g)): GI of 52, GL of 8, Net carb= 20g

▦ Pea Powder, (1 tbsp (8g)): GI of 22, GL of 1, Net carb= 4g

▦ Pea Puree, (½ cup (125g)): GI of 45, GL of 5, Net carb= 16g

▦ Peppers, hot chili, green, raw, (1 pepper (14g)): GI of 30-35, GL of 1, Net carb= 1g

▤ Peppers, hot chili, red, raw, (1 pepper (45g)): GI of 30-35, GL of 1, Net carb= 2g

▤ Peppers, Hungarian, raw, (1 cup (125g)): GI of 15-20, GL of 1, Net carb= 5g

▤ Peppers, jalapeno, raw, (1 pepper (14g)): GI of 30-35, GL of 1, Net carb= 0.6g

▤ Peppers, serrano, raw, (1 pepper (18g)): GI of 30-35, GL of 1, Net carb= 1g

▤ Peppers, sweet, green, raw, (1 cup (149g)): GI of 15-20, GL of 2, Net carb= 6g

▤ Peppers, sweet, red, raw, (1 cup (149g)): GI of 15-20, GL of 2, Net carb= 6g

▤ Peppers, sweet, yellow, raw, (1 cup (149g)): GI of 15-20, GL of 2, Net carb= 6g

▤ Pesto, (1 tbsp (15g)): GI of 15, GL of 0, Net carb= 1g

▤ Plantain Chips, (1 oz (28g)): GI of 50, GL of 7, Net carb= 15g

▤ Potato Chips, (1 oz (28g)): GI of 56, GL of 8, Net carb= 15g

▤ Pumpkin Cooked , (1 cup (245g)): GI of 15, GL of 3, Net carb= 12g

▤ Pumpkin flowers, raw, (1 cup (18g)): GI of 15-20, GL of 1, Net carb= 0.5g

▤ Pumpkin Juice, (1 cup (240ml)): GI of 15, GL of 3, Net carb= 12g

▤ Pumpkin leaves, raw, (1 cup (33g)): GI of 15-20, GL of 1, Net carb= 0.6g

▤ Pumpkin Powder, (1 tbsp (6g)): GI of 15, GL of 0, Net carb= 2g

▤ Pumpkin Puree, (1/2 cup (125g)): GI of 15, GL of 2, Net carb= 10g

▤ Purslane, raw, (1 cup (43g)): GI of 15-20, GL of 1, Net carb= 0.7g

▤ Radicchio, (1 cup (40g)): GI of 15, GL of 0, Net carb= 1g

▤ Radish Chips, (1 oz (28g)): GI of 15, GL of 1, Net carb= 6g

▤ Radish Juice, (1 cup (240ml)): GI of 15, GL of 1, Net carb= 6g

▤ Radish, (1 cup (116g)): GI of 15, GL of 0, Net carb= 2g

▤ Red Bell Pepper Powder, (1 tbsp (6g)): GI of 15, GL of 0, Net carb= 2g

▤ Red Cabbage Juice, (1 cup (240ml)): GI of 15, GL of 1, Net carb= 9g

▤ Rhubarb Cooked, (1 cup (122g)): GI of 15, GL of 1, Net carb= 5g

▤ Roasted Red Pepper Dip, (2 tbsp (30g)): GI of 15, GL of 1, Net carb= 3g

▤ Rutabaga Cooked Bolied Drained, (½ cup (85g)): GI of 72, GL of 5, Net carb= 8g

▤ Salsa, (2 tbsp (30g)): GI of 25, GL of 1, Net carb= 2g

▤ Salsify Cooked Boiled With Salt Drained, (1 cup (133g)): GI of 30-35, GL of 3, Net carb= 8g

▤ Salsify Cooked Boiled Without Salt Drained, (1 cup (133g)): GI of 30-35, GL of 3, Net carb= 8g

▤ Salsify, raw, (1 cup (133g)): GI of 30-35, GL of 3, Net carb= 8g

▤ Seaweed, agar, raw, (1 cup (40g)): GI of 15-20, GL of 1, Net carb= 1g

▤ Seaweed, irishmoss, raw, (1 cup (40g)): GI of 15-20, GL of 1, Net carb= 2g

▤ Seaweed, kelp, raw, (1 cup (36g)): GI of 15-20, GL of 1, Net carb= 1g

▤ Seaweed, laver, raw, (1 cup (25g)): GI of 15-20, GL of 1, Net carb= 1g

⊞ Seaweed, spirulina, raw, (1 tbsp (7g)): GI of 15-20, GL of 1, Net carb= 0.3g

⊞ Seaweed, wakame, raw, (1 cup (10g)): GI of 15-20, GL of 1, Net carb= 0.5g

⊞ Sesbania flower, raw, (1 cup (25g)): GI of 15-20, GL of 1, Net carb= 1g

⊞ Shallot, (1 tbsp (10g)): GI of 15, GL of 0.3, Net carb= 2g

⊞ Snap Pea Crisps, (1 oz (28g)): GI of 45, GL of 3, Net carb= 8g

⊞ Sorrel, (1 cup (29g)): GI of 15, GL of 0, Net carb= 1g

⊞ Soybean sprouts, (1 cup (172g)): GI of 20, GL of 3, Net carb= 10g

⊞ Soybeans, (1 cup (172g)): GI of 20, GL of 3, Net carb= 10g

⊞ Spaghetti Squash, (1 cup (155g)): GI of 15, GL of 1, Net carb= 7g

⊞ Spinach and Ginger Juice, (1 cup (240ml)): GI of 15, GL of 1, Net carb= 7g

⊞ Spinach Chips, (1 oz (28g)): GI of 15, GL of 1, Net carb= 6g

⊞ Spinach Cooked, (1 cup (180g)): GI of 15, GL of 0.6, Net carb= 4g

⊞ Spinach Dip, (2 tbsp (30g)): GI of 15, GL of 1, Net carb= 2g

⊞ Spinach Juice, (1 cup (240ml)): GI of 15, GL of 1, Net carb= 5g

⊞ Spinach Powder, (1 tbsp (7g)): GI of 15, GL of 0.1, Net carb= 1g

⊞ Spinach Puree, (1/2 cup (125g)): GI of 15, GL of 0.1, Net carb= 1g

⊞ Squash Acorn, Cooked , (½ cup (102g)): GI of 75, GL of 7.5, Net carb= 15g

⊞ Squash Butternut, Cooked , (½ cup (102g)): GI of 51, GL of 8, Net carb= 21g

⊞ Squash Spaghetti, Cooked , (1 cup (155g)): GI of 15, GL of 1, Net carb= 7g

▤ Squash, winter, acorn, raw, (1 cup (140g)): GI of 40-45, GL of 6, Net carb= 15g

▤ Squash, winter, butternut, raw, (1 cup (140g)): GI of 45-50, GL of 6, Net carb= 13g

▤ Squash, winter, hubbard, raw, (1 cup (116g)): GI of 40-45, GL of 5, Net carb= 11g

▤ Squash, winter, spaghetti, raw, (1 cup (101g)): GI of 15-20, GL of 1, Net carb= 5g

▤ Sweet Potato Chips, (1 oz (28g)): GI of 54, GL of 9, Net carb= 16g

▤ Sweet potato leaves, raw, (1 cup (28g)): GI of 15-20, GL of 1, Net carb= 1g

▤ Sweet Potato Noodles, (½ cup (70g)): GI of 63, GL of 4.5, Net carb= 11g

▤ Sweet Potato Powder, (1 tbsp (8g)): GI of 63, GL of 3, Net carb= 6g

▤ Swiss Chard, (1 cup (175g)): GI of 15, GL of 1, Net carb= 4g

▤ Tapenade, (1 tbsp (15g)): GI of 15, GL of 0, Net carb= 1g

▤ Taro leaves, raw, (1 cup (28g)): GI of 15-20, GL of 1, Net carb= 1g

▤ Taro Root Chips, (1 oz (28g)): GI of 55, GL of 7, Net carb= 14g

▤ Taro shoots, raw, (1 cup (84g)): GI of 15-20, GL of 1, Net carb= 2g

▤ Taro, Tahitian, raw, (½ cup (104g)): GI of 50-55, GL of 9, Net carb= 12.5g

▤ Tomatillo, (1 cup (132g)): GI of 15, GL of 1, Net carb= 4g

▤ Tomato Juice, (1 cup (240ml)): GI of 38, GL of 5, Net carb= 10g

▤ Tomato Powder, (1 tbsp (7g)): GI of 38, GL of 1, Net carb= 3g

▤ Tomato Puree, (1/2 cup (125g)): GI of 38, GL of 2, Net carb= 7g

▤ Tomato, chopped , (1 cup (180g)): GI of 15, GL of 1, Net carb= 5g

▤ Turmeric Juice, (1 tbsp (15ml)): GI of 15, GL of 0, Net carb= 1g

▤ Turnip Noodles, (1 cup (130g)): GI of 15, GL of 1, Net carb= 4g

▤ Turnip, (1 cup (156g)): GI of 62, GL of 4, Net carb= 8g

▤ Vinespinach, (basella), raw, (1 cup (44g)): GI of 15-20, GL of 1, Net carb= 0.8g

▤ Wasabi, root, raw, (1 tbsp (10g)): GI of 15-20, GL of 1, Net carb= 1g

▤ Waterchestnuts, chinese, raw, (1 cup (150g)): GI of 60, GL of 9, Net carb= 24g

▤ Watercress Juice, (1 cup (240ml)): GI of 15, GL of 1, Net carb= 4g

▤ Watercress, (1 cup (34g)): GI of 15, GL of 0, Net carb= 0g

▤ Wax Beans, (1 cup (125g)): GI of 15, GL of 1, Net carb= 5g

▤ Wheatgrass Juice, (1 ounce (30ml)): GI of 15, GL of 0, Net carb= 1g

▤ Winged bean leaves, raw, (1 cup (42g)): GI of 15-20, GL of 1, Net carb= 0.7g

▤ Winged bean tuber, raw, (1 cup (94g)): GI of 35-40, GL of 6, Net carb= 17g

▤ Yardlong bean, raw, (1 cup (100g)): GI of 15-20, GL of 1, Net carb= 5.5g

▤ Zucchini Chips, (1 oz (28g)): GI of 15, GL of 2, Net carb= 12g

▤ Zucchini Juice, (1 cup (240ml)): GI of 15, GL of 2, Net carb= 11g

▤ Zucchini Noodles (Zoodles), (1 cup (120g)): GI of 15, GL of 2, Net carb= 4g

▤ Zucchini Powder, (1 tbsp (7g)): GI of 15, GL of 1, Net carb= 4g

▤ Zucchini, baby (courgette), raw, (1 cup (127g)): GI of 15, GL of 1, Net carb= 3g

▤ Zucchini, (1 cup (124g)): GI of 15, GL of 2, Net carb= 6g

* * *

MEDIUM GLYCEMIC LOAD FOODS A-Z

In the DiabeteBalance Diet, we prioritize a strategic approach that empowers you to make informed dietary choices. While we emphasize foods with a low glycemic load as the adequate choice for optimally managing type 2 diabetes, we understand the need for variety and occasional indulgences.

Thus, we also provide comprehensive information on foods that fall within the medium glycemic load category. These are not the optimal option for regular consumption, but we believe in giving you a complete understanding of your options to help you navigate your food choices.

For each food item in this medium category, we present key details including typical serving size, Glycemic Index (GI), Glycemic Load (GL), and Net Carbohydrates. Armed with this information, you can make more conscious decisions even when you decide to consume these foods on occasion.

However, it's crucial to remember that portion control is vital when indulging in these foods. While they can be tolerated occasionally, we highly recommend reducing the standard serving size to ensure that your intake stays below 15 grams of net carbohydrates. This approach will help you maintain better blood sugar control while still allowing some flexibility in your diet.

* * *

▤ Cassava, Cooked , (½ cup (110g)): GI of 46, GL of 18, Net carb= 39g

▤ Corn, sweet, white, raw, (½ cup (82g)): GI of 60, GL of 11.4, Net carb= 19g

▤ Corn, sweet, yellow, raw, (½ cup (82g)): GI of 60, GL of 11.4, Net carb= 19g

▤ Mountain yam, hawaii, raw, (½ cup (82g)): GI of 58, GL of 11, Net carb= 18g

▤ Potato, Cooked , (½ cup (105g)): GI of 78, GL of 11, Net carb= 15g

▤ Potatoes, flesh and skin, raw, (1 medium (213g)): GI of 60-65, GL of 18, Net carb= 33g

▤ Sweet Potato Puree, (½ cup cup (125g)): GI of 63, GL of 12, Net carb= 24g

▤ Sweet Potato, Cooked, (½ cup cup (125g)): GI of 63, GL of 11.3, Net carb= 18g

PART VI
THE WORST FOODS TO EAT

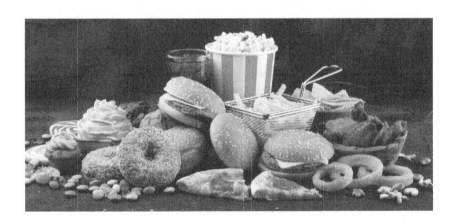

UNDERSTANDING FOODS TO EXCLUDE IN THE T2D REVERSAL DIET

In the framework of the DiabeteBalance Diet, specific foods can present challenges to the optimal management of Type 2 Diabetes. Understanding the attributes that define these unfavorable food choices is key to adherence. Here are the criteria that characterize these foods:

- **High Glycemic Load (GL):** Foods with elevated GL provoke immediate and pronounced elevations in blood sugar, stemming from the quantity and type of carbohydrates they contain. Regular consumption of these items can encourage insulin resistance, thereby obstructing ideal T2D control.
- **Highly Processed Foods:** Even if a food item's GL is classified as low or medium, excessive processing might render it detrimental. Unhealthy additives, excessive salt, sugars, and unhealthy fats often accompany these foods, potentially leading to weight gain and inflammation. Such consequences can adversely impact blood sugar regulation and overall well-being.
- **Deviation from Mediterranean Diet Principles:** Non-alignment with the principles of the Mediterranean diet

constitutes another unfavorable aspect. This dietary approach emphasizes whole or minimally processed foods, including fruits, vegetables, olive oil, whole grains, lean proteins, and beneficial fats. Foods contrary to these principles, such as those heavily processed or lacking in nutritional value, can impede T2D management.

- **Contradiction with 2020-2025 Dietary Guidelines for Americans:** Foods that do not adhere to these guidelines are also problematic. These guidelines advocate the consumption of nutrient-dense foods that are affluent in vital vitamins, minerals, and other beneficial substances but are calorie-efficient. Foods replete with added sugars, unhealthy fats, and sodium fall short of these criteria.

Armed with this indispensable insight, subsequent chapters will delve into distinct food categories like vegetables, fruits and derivatives, meats, beverages, grains, etc. Each will furnish a detailed roster of non-compliant foods, encompassing serving sizes, GI, GL, and net carbohydrate values, as applicable. The discourse will also cover foods with low or medium GL that clash with other foundational diet principles, accentuating the multifaceted nature of dietary management in diabetes.

Though the DiabeteBalance Diet primarily discourages non-compliant foods, sporadic indulgence is permissible, provided meticulous monitoring of portion sizes and frequencies. Adhering to a daily GL goal, ideally within the threshold of 50, constitutes an essential facet of efficacious diabetes management.

The mastery of portion size is pivotal when dining externally as well. Choices at restaurants should preferably align with Mediterranean diet standards, with vigilant scrutiny of portion sizes and supplementary ingredients. Fast-food and typical American-style restaurants may serve dishes that markedly deviate from these guidelines. In constrained situations, selecting the healthiest available option and contemplating sharing or saving a portion for later is advisable.

Navigating non-compliant foods can be intricate, but perseverance and an educated methodology can facilitate this component of diet management. Strategies such as scrutinizing labels, pre-planning meals, practicing mindful eating, and intelligent substitutions can aid in surmounting these obstacles.

Persistently opting for healthier alternatives will foster habits conducive to the DiabeteBalance Diet, rendering the distinction between compliant and non-compliant foods intuitive. Nonetheless, recognizing the uniqueness of every individual's journey is vital. Seeking professional guidance and progressing incrementally towards dietary goals is not only acceptable but often beneficial.

BREADS AND BAKED PRODUCTS

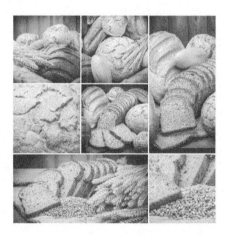

While bread and baked products can be integral to a balanced diet for individuals with Type 2 Diabetes (T2D), there are circumstances in which certain bread and baked products may conflict with the principles of the DiabeteBalance Diet.

These non-compliant products typically fall afoul of guidelines due to factors such as a high glycemic index (GI), excessive carbohydrate content, the presence of artificial additives, unhealthy fats, high sodium levels, or additional problematic elements. The consumption of these bread and baked products can adversely impact blood sugar regulation, impede overall health, and obstruct the targeted objectives of T2D management.

Bread and baked products that diverge from the DiabeteBalance Diet principles encompass:

- **White Bread:** Made from refined grains stripped of their fiber and nutrients, white bread has a high GI, resulting in quick and significant increases in blood sugar levels.
- **Sweetened or Flavored Breads:** Examples include cinnamon raisin bread, sweet fruit breads, or sweet rolls, which can escalate carbohydrate and sugar consumption, leading to blood sugar elevation.
- **Pastries and Sweet Baked Goods:** Items such as croissants, doughnuts, muffins, and sweet rolls, rich in butter, sugar, and refined flour, can be calorie-dense and carbohydrate-heavy.
- **Sweet Breads and Rolls:** Products like cinnamon rolls and danishes, which are typically high in sugar and low in fiber.
- **Bagels:** Even a single bagel can be equivalent to several slices of bread in carbohydrates, potentially triggering blood sugar spikes.
- **Biscuits and Scones:** Often high in unhealthy fats and deficient in fiber, these are incompatible with the DiabeteBalance Diet.
- **Flavored and Sweetened Cornbread:** While traditional cornbread may be acceptable, variants with added sweeteners may not align with the diet's guidelines.
- **Sugary Muffins and Cakes:** These include muffins, cupcakes, cakes, and cake-like desserts made with refined flour, sugars, and high-fat ingredients, detrimental to both blood sugar control and weight management.
- **Sugar-Laden Cookies and Pastries:** Such cookies and

pastries made with refined flour and abundant added sugars can imbalance blood sugar and contribute to overeating.

- **High-Carb Crackers and Pretzels:** Often made from refined grains, these snacks are typically high in carbohydrates and low in fiber, causing rapid blood sugar elevation.
- **Gluten-Free Products with Added Sugars and Fats:** Some gluten-free bread and baked goods may contain extra sugars and fats to improve texture and taste, making them less suitable for the DiabeteBalance Diet.

In the subsequent section of this chapter, an exhaustive list of non-compliant foods associated with the DiabeteBalance Diet is provided. These tables contain meticulous details such as serving size, Glycemic Index (GI), Glycemic Load (GL), and Net Carbohydrates for each item. Such metrics are vital when a food item's incongruence is tied to a high glycemic load or substantial carbohydrate content.

HIGH GL and/or HIGH CARB FOOD

Baguette, (1 serving, 50g): GI of 95, GL of 23, Net carb= 25g

Almond Poppy Seed Bread (store bought), (1 serving, 50g): GI of High, GL of High, Net carb= Varies

Apple Cinnamon Muffins (store bought), (1 serving, 50g): GI of High, GL of High, Net carb= Varies

Banana Bread (store bought), (1 serving, 50g): GI of High, GL of High, Net carb= Varies

Blueberry Muffins (store bought), (1 serving, 50g): GI of High, GL of High, Net carb= Varies

Carrot Muffins (store bought), (1 serving, 50g): GI of High, GL of High, Net carb= Varies

▤ Cherry Pie, (1 slice, 125g): GI of 70, GL of 21, Net carb= 31g

▤ Chocolate Chip Muffins (store bought), (1 serving, 50g): GI of High, GL of High, Net carb= Varies

▤ Chocolate Pecan Pie, (1 slice, 125g): GI of 55, GL of 23.1, Net carb= 42g

▤ Cinnamon Swirl Bread (store bought), (1 serving, 50g): GI of High, GL of High, Net carb= Varies

▤ Coffee Cake (store bought), (1 serving, 50g): GI of High, GL of High, Net carb= Varies

▤ Commercially-prepared cakes with added frosting, fillings, or glazes., (1 serving, 50g): GI of High, GL of High, Net carb= Varies

▤ commercially-prepared cookies with added frosting, fillings, or glazes., (1 serving, 50g): GI of High, GL of High, Net carb= Varies

▤ Commercially-prepared cupcakes with added frosting, fillings, or glazes., (1 serving, 50g): GI of High, GL of High, Net carb= Varies

▤ Cranberry Orange Bread (store bought), (1 serving, 50g): GI of High, GL of High, Net carb= Varies

▤ Danish Pastry, (1 medium, 84g): GI of 59, GL of 22, Net carb= 37g

▤ Double Chocolate Muffins (store bought), (1 serving, 50g): GI of High, GL of High, Net carb= Varies

▤ Hummingbird Cake, (1 slice, 80g): GI of 67, GL of 21, Net carb= 37g

▤ Key Lime Pie, (1 serving, 50g): GI of High, GL of High, Net carb= Varies

▤ Lemon Meringue Pie, (1 serving, 50g): GI of High, GL of High, Net carb= Varies

▤ Lemon Poppy Seed Muffins (store bought), (1 serving, 50g): GI of High, GL of High, Net carb= Varies

▤ Mississippi Mud Pie, (1 slice, 100g): GI of 60, GL of 24, Net carb= 30g

▤ Opera Cake, (1 slice, 80g): GI of 65, GL of 23, Net carb= 28g

▤ Peach Muffins (store bought), (1 serving, 50g): GI of High, GL of High, Net carb= Varies

▤ Pecan Pie, (1 slice, 125g): GI of 50, GL of 26, Net carb= 41g

▤ Pretzels (store bought), (1 serving, 50g): GI of High, GL of High, Net carb= Varies

▤ Pumpkin Bread (store bought), (1 serving, 50g): GI of High, GL of High, Net carb= Varies

▤ Pumpkin Pie, (1 slice, 125g): GI of 75, GL of 22, Net carb= 30g

▤ Raspberry Streusel Bread (store bought), (1 serving, 50g): GI of High, GL of High, Net carb= Varies

▤ Rice Cakes, (1 serving, 50g): GI of High, GL of High, Net carb= Varies

▤ Vanilla Cake, (1 slice, 100g): GI of 65, GL of 22, Net carb= 42g

▤ Waffles with sugary syrups, (1 serving, 50g): GI of High, GL of High, Net carb= Varies

▤ Zucchini Bread (store bought), (1 serving, 50g): GI of High, GL of High, Net carb= Varies

LEGUMES AND PULSES

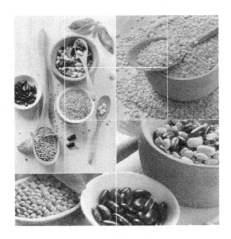

While legumes and pulses generally benefit individuals with T2D due to their high fiber content and blood sugar regulation properties, it's critical to recognize that certain legume and pulse-based products may conflict with the principles of the DiabeteBalance Diet.

Non-compliant legume-based products can harbor high sugar content, excessive carbohydrates, artificial additives, unhealthy fats, or increased sodium levels. The consumption of these products can negatively impact blood sugar control, overall health, and obstruct T2D management goals. Therefore, understanding the nutritional composition of legume-based products is key, and choosing those that harmonize with the DiabeteBalance Diet is recommended.

- **Canned Beans:** These often contain added sugars and sodium. The preferred choices would be low-sodium, low-sugar varieties or homemade versions.
- **Refried Beans:** Certain brands or types of refried beans pose concerns due to unhealthy fats, high sodium, or potentially added sugars. Some examples of non-compliant refried beans include:
- **Canned Refried Beans with Added Fats:** Some versions are cooked with extra fats, often unhealthy, contributing to calorie surplus and weight gain.
- **Canned Refried Beans with High Sodium:** Sodium, added for taste and preservation, can escalate blood pressure, a common issue associated with diabetes.
- **Canned Refried Beans with Added Sugars:** Some brands may add sugars, leading to increased blood glucose levels, albeit this is less common.
- **Restaurant-Served Refried Beans:** Restaurants might prepare refried beans with large amounts of unhealthy fats or high-sodium or sugar ingredients.
- **Refried Beans with Full-Fat Cheese:** Cheese often accompanies refried beans, and full-fat versions can boost calorie and saturated fat intake.
- **Sweetened Lentil-Based Snacks or Desserts:** These include products like sweetened lentil-based pastries, desserts, or snack bars that can have added sugars and unhealthy fats.
- **Fried or Salted Nuts and Seeds:** While nuts and seeds are technically legumes, fried versions or those with added salt can be high in unhealthy fats and sodium.
- **Canned Chickpeas with Added Sugars or Fats:** Some brands might add extra sugars or fats to their canned

chickpeas, making them less suitable for the DiabeteBalance Diet.

- **Processed Soy Products:** Certain soy products, such as processed soy meats or snacks, can contain added sugars, unhealthy fats, and high sodium levels.

FLAVORED REFRIED BEANS:

Some versions of refried beans come with additional flavorings or ingredients, which can add to their sugar, fat, and sodium content.

The following is a list of items that are not suitable for individuals with diabetes:

Black Bean Refried Beans ▤ Cheesy Refried Beans ▤ Creamy Refried Beans ▤ Cuban-Style Refried Beans ▤ Frijoles Charros (Refried Beans with Bacon and Chorizo) ▤ Green Chile Refried Beans ▤ Guajillo Refried Beans ▤ Instant Pot Refried Beans ▤ Jalapeño Refried Beans ▤ Mexican-Style Refried Beans ▤ Pinto Bean Refried Beans ▤ Ranch-Style Refried Beans ▤ Refried Beans with Avocado ▤ Refried Beans with Bacon ▤ Refried Beans with Caramelized Onions ▤ Refried Beans with Cheddar Cheese ▤ Refried Beans with Cheese ▤ Refried Beans with Chipotle Powder ▤ Refried Beans with Chorizo ▤ Refried Beans with Cilantro ▤ Refried Beans with Corn ▤ Refried Beans with Cumin ▤ Refried Beans with Epazote ▤ Refried Beans with Epazote and Cumin ▤ Refried Beans with Garlic ▤ Refried Beans with Green Onions ▤ Refried Beans with Ground Beef ▤ Refried Beans with Guacamole ▤ Refried Beans with Guajillo Chili Powder ▤ Refried Beans with Jalapeños ▤ Refried Beans with Lime ▤ Refried Beans with Mexican Crema ▤ Refried Beans with Onion ▤ Refried Beans with Oregano ▤ Refried Beans with Paprika ▤ Refried Beans with Pico de Gallo ▤ Refried Beans with Queso Fresco ▤ Refried Beans with Red Pepper Flakes ▤ Refried Beans with Salsa ▤ Refried Beans with Serrano Peppers ▤ Refried Beans with Smoked

Paprika ▤ Refried Beans with Sour Cream ▤ Refried Beans with Tomatoes ▤ Refried Black Beans with Cilantro ▤ Slow Cooker Refried Beans ▤ Smoky Chipotle Refried Beans ▤ Spiced Refried Beans ▤ Spicy Refried Beans ▤ Traditional Refried Beans ▤ Vegan Refried Beans

---

SWEETENED OR FLAVORED LEGUMES:

Some pre-packaged legumes and pulses can have added sugars or high-sodium sauces and seasonings. For example, canned chickpeas in a sweetened sauce or black beans in a high-sodium taco mix might not be the best options.

The following is a list of items that are not suitable for individuals with diabetes:

▤ Canned Legumes in Barbecue Sauce ▤ Canned Legumes in Blueberry Sauce ▤ Canned Legumes in Bourbon Sauce ▤ Canned Legumes in Brown Sugar Glaze ▤ Canned Legumes in Coconut Curry Sauce ▤ Canned Legumes in Hoisin Sauce ▤ Canned Legumes in Honey Lime Sauce ▤ Canned Legumes in Honey Mustard Sauce ▤ Canned Legumes in Mango Habanero Sauce ▤ Canned Legumes in Mango Sauce ▤ Canned Legumes in Maple BBQ Sauce ▤ Canned Legumes in Orange Glaze ▤ Canned Legumes in Peach Sauce ▤ Canned Legumes in Pineapple Sauce ▤ Canned Legumes in Pineapple Teriyaki Sauce ▤ Canned Legumes in Raspberry Sauce ▤ Canned Legumes in Strawberry Sauce ▤ Canned Legumes in Sweet and Sour Sauce ▤ Canned Legumes in Sweet and Spicy Sauce ▤ Canned Legumes in Sweet and Tangy Sauce ▤ Canned Legumes in Sweet Barbecue Sauce ▤ Canned Legumes in Sweet Basil Sauce ▤ Canned Legumes in Sweet Buffalo Sauce ▤ Canned Legumes in Sweet Cajun Sauce ▤ Canned Legumes in Sweet Chili Sauce ▤ Canned Legumes in Sweet Chipotle Sauce ▤ Canned Legumes in Sweet Cilantro Lime Sauce ▤ Canned Legumes in Sweet Curry Sauce ▤ Canned Legumes in Sweet Garlic Sauce ▦ Canned Legumes in Sweet Ginger Sauce ▦ Canned Legumes in Sweet Herb Sauce ▦ Canned Legumes in Sweet Lemon Sauce ▦ Canned Legumes in Sweet Mustard Sauce ▦ Canned Legumes in Sweet Onion Sauce ▦ Canned Legumes in Sweet Paprika Sauce ▦ Canned Legumes in Sweet Pesto Sauce ▦ Canned Legumes in Sweet Ranch Sauce ▦ Canned Legumes in Sweet Sesame Sauce ▦ Canned Legumes in Sweet Soy Sauce ▦ Canned Legumes in Sweet Sriracha Sauce ▦ Canned Legumes in Sweet Sun-Dried Tomato Sauce ▦ Canned Legumes in Sweet Worcestershire Sauce ▦ Canned Legumes in Tomato Sauce with Added Sugar ▦ Canned Sweetened Baked Beans ▦ Flavored Canned Black Beans in Sauce ▦ Honey-Glazed Canned Lentils ▦ Maple Syrup Canned Navy Beans ▦ Sweet Chili Sauce Canned Kidney Beans ▦ Sweetened Canned Chickpeas ▦ Teriyaki-Flavored Canned Edamame

PROCESSED PULSES:

Products made from pulses, such as certain types of crackers or snacks, usually contain other high-carb ingredients and are lower in fiber.

▦ Black Bean-based Breakfast Burritos with Added Flour Tortillas ▦ Black Bean-based Cookies with Added Refined Wheat Flour ▦ Black Bean-based Donuts with Added Wheat Flour ▦ Black Bean-based Pretzels with Added Wheat Flour ▦ Black Bean-based Rice Cakes with Added Grain Fillers ▦ Black Bean-based Veggie Sausages with Added Fillers ▦ Black Bean-based Waffles with Added Starches ▦ Chickpea-based Bread with Added Wheat Flour ▦ Chickpea-based Breakfast Cereals with Added Artificial Sweeteners ▦ Chickpea-based Breakfast Cereals with Added Sugars ▦ Chickpea-based Cereal Bars with Added Artificial Colors ▦ Chickpea-based Cereal Bars with Added Sugars ▦ Chickpea-based Chips with Added Antioxidants ▦ Chickpea-based Cookies with Added Trans Fats ▦ Chickpea-based

Crackers with Added Hydrogenated Oils ▦ Chickpea-based Crackers with Added Vegetable Oils ▦ Chickpea-based Crackers with Added Wheat Flour ▦ Chickpea-based Donuts with Added Artificial Coloring ▦ Chickpea-based Pancake Mix with Added Artificial Sweeteners ▦ Chickpea-based Pancake Mix with Added Sugar Substitutes ▦ Chickpea-based Pasta with Added Gluten ▦ Chickpea-based Pita Chips with Added Artificial Sweeteners ▦ Chickpea-based Pita Chips with Added White Flour ▦ Chickpea-based Pizza Crust with Added Wheat Grains ▦ Chickpea-based Pretzels with Added Preservatives ▦ Chickpea-based Snack Bars with Added High-Fructose Corn Syrup ▦ Chickpea-based Tortilla Chips with Added Cornmeal ▦ Chickpea-based Tortilla Chips with Added MSG ▦ Lentil-based Bread with Added Dough Conditioners ▦ Lentil-based Chips with Added Artificial Flavorings ▦ Lentil-based Chips with Added Maltodextrin ▦ Lentil-based Chips with Added Potato Starch ▦ Lentil-based Crackers with Added Emulsifiers ▦ Lentil-based Granola Bars with Added Artificial Preservatives ▦ Lentil-based Granola Bars with Added Sweeteners ▦ Lentil-based Muffins with Added Artificial Flavors ▦ Lentil-based Muffins with Added Refined Flours ▦ Lentil-based Pancake Mix with Added All-Purpose Flour ▦ Lentil-based Pasta with Added Enriched Wheat Flour ▦ Lentil-based Pizza Crust with Added Yeast Enhancers ▦ Lentil-based Puffs with Added Artificial Colorings ▦ Lentil-based Rice Cakes with Added Artificial Additives ▦ Lentil-based Snack Mix with Added High-Fructose Corn Syrup ▦ Lentil-based Snack Mix with Added Wheat Cereals ▦ Lentil-based Veggie Burgers with Added Bread Crumbs ▦ Lentil-based Waffles with Added Cornstarch ▦ Lentil-based Waffles with Added Fillers ▦ Pea-based Puffs with Added Rice Cereal ▦ Split Pea-based Crackers with Added Wheat Flour ▦ Split Pea-based Pasta with Added Semolina Flour

Remember to always consider the nutritional content of any legume or pulse-based product and ensure it adheres to the DiabeteBalance

Diet principles. The next section in this chapter will provide a comprehensive list of non-compliant legume-based foods along with their serving size, Glycemic Index (GI), Glycemic Load (GL), and Net Carbohydrates, assisting you in your healthy meal planning efforts.

▤ Adzuki Beans, Canned, Regular: Non-compliant foods

▤ Black Beans, Canned, Regular: Non-compliant foods

▤ Black-eyed Peas, Canned, Regular: Non-compliant foods

▤ Butter Beans, Canned, Regular: Non-compliant foods

▤ Cannellini Beans, Canned, Regular: Non-compliant foods

▤ Cranberry Beans, Canned, Regular: Non-compliant foods

▤ Fava Beans, Canned, Regular: Non-compliant foods

▤ Garbanzo Beans, Canned, Regular: Non-compliant foods

▤ Great Northern Beans, Canned, Regular: Non-compliant foods

▤ Green Snap Beans, Canned, Regular: Non-compliant foods

▤ Green String Beans, Canned, Regular: Non-compliant foods

▤ Highly processed Bean-based "Bacon": Non-compliant foods

▤ Highly processed Bean-based "Chicken": Non-compliant foods

▤ Highly processed Bean-based "Corned Beef": Non-compliant foods

▤ Highly processed Bean-based "Ham": Non-compliant foods

▤ Highly processed Bean-based "Pastrami": Non-compliant foods

▤ Highly processed Bean-based "Pepperoni": Non-compliant foods

▤ Highly processed Bean-based "Roast Beef": Non-compliant foods

▤ Highly processed Bean-based "Salami": Non-compliant foods

▤ Highly processed Bean-based "Turkey": Non-compliant foods

▤ Highly processed Veggie Burgers: Non-compliant foods

▤ Kidney Beans, Canned, Regular: Non-compliant foods

▤ Lentils, Canned, Regular: Non-compliant foods

▤ Lima Beans, Canned, Regular: Non-compliant foods

▤ Mung Beans, Canned, Regular: Non-compliant foods

▤ Navy Beans, Canned, Regular: Non-compliant foods

▤ Pinto Beans, Canned, Regular: Non-compliant foods

▤ Red Beans, Canned, Regular: Non-compliant foods

▤ Soybeans, Canned, Regular: Non-compliant foods

▤ Sweetened Azuki Beans, (1 serving, 50g): GI value= High, GL value= High, Net carb= Varies

▤ Sweetened Black-Eyed Peas, (1 serving, 50g): GI value= High, GL value= High, Net carb= Varies

▤ Sweetened Cannellini Beans, (1 serving, 50g): GI value= High, GL value= High, Net carb= Varies

▤ Sweetened Chickpeas, (1 serving, 50g): GI value= High, GL value= High, Net carb= Varies

▤ Sweetened Great Northern Beans, (1 serving, 50g): GI value= High, GL value= High, Net carb= Varies

▤ Sweetened Kidney Beans, (1 serving, 50g): GI value= High, GL value= High, Net carb= Varies

▤ Sweetened Lentils, (1 serving, 50g): GI value= High, GL value= High, Net carb= Varies

▤ Sweetened Lima Beans, (1 serving, 50g): GI value= High, GL value= High, Net carb= Varies

▤ Sweetened Mung Beans, (1 serving, 50g): GI value= High, GL value= High, Net carb= Varies

▤ Sweetened Navy Beans, (1 serving, 50g): GI value= High, GL value= High, Net carb= Varies

▤ Sweetened Pinto Beans, (1 serving, 50g): GI value= High, GL value= High, Net carb= Varies

▤ Sweetened Red Beans, (1 serving, 50g): GI value= High, GL value= High, Net carb= Varies

▤ Sweetened Soybeans, (1 serving, 50g): GI value= High, GL value= High, Net carb= Varies

BEVERAGES AND DRINKS

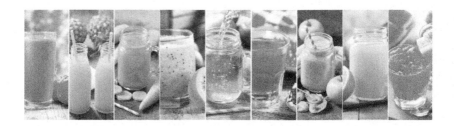

A wide range of beverages, though often tempting, regularly conflict with the principles of the DiabeteBalance Diet, which incorporates Glycemic Load (GL) guidelines, the Mediterranean Diet, the 2020-2025 Dietary Guidelines for Americans, and 14 principles of a healthy, balanced diet.

Non-compliant beverages can possess high sugar content, excessive carbohydrates, artificial additives, unhealthy fats, or increased sodium levels. Consumption of such drinks can negatively impact blood sugar control, overall health, and impede T2D management goals.

- **Sugary Drinks and Sodas:** High in added sugars and devoid of nutritional value, these drinks can spike blood sugar levels rapidly and significantly contribute to excessive caloric intake, exacerbating T2D. They directly contravene the low GL, balanced nutrient intake, and limited sugar intake principles of the DiabeteBalance Diet.

- **Fruit Juices:** Whether freshly squeezed or labeled as 100% juice, fruit juices are problematic due to their concentrated natural sugars and absence of fiber found in whole fruit. They can cause rapid blood glucose increases and don't satiate as effectively as whole fruits, hence conflicting with the balanced glycemic response and sufficient fiber intake principles fundamental to the DiabeteBalance Diet.

- **Alcoholic Beverages:** Excessive consumption can contribute to weight gain and blood sugar instability. Moreover, they can interfere with some diabetes medications, impeding effective T2D management. Moderate wine consumption, integral to the MedDiet, is the key. However, not all alcoholic beverages are recommended.

- **Sweetened Teas and Coffees:** Tea and coffee are not problematic per se, but the addition of sugars, syrups, and creamers can make them less suitable. These additives can cause blood glucose spikes and contribute to weight gain, conflicting with the low GL and low added sugars guidelines of the DiabeteBalance Diet.

- **Energy and Sports Drinks:** These beverages, often loaded with sugars and caffeine, can cause a quick surge and subsequent drop in blood sugar levels, presenting problems for T2D management. They're typically high in calories and offer little nutritional benefit, hence conflicting with the principles of balanced nutrient intake and controlled caloric intake.

- **Flavored Waters:** Some bottled waters come with added sugars or artificial sweeteners that can disrupt blood sugar control and are inconsistent with the DiabeteBalance Diet principles.

- **Milkshakes and Sweetened Dairy Drinks:** These drinks are typically high in sugar, calories, and sometimes unhealthy fats, all of which can hinder blood sugar control and weight management.

Choose water, unsweetened teas, and occasionally moderate amounts of coffee (without sweeteners or unhealthy creamers) instead of these drinks. If you consume alcohol, moderation is essential, with wine or light beer being generally the best options. The goal is to avoid rapid blood glucose spikes and unnecessary caloric intake, while maintaining a balance of nutrients in line with the DiabeteBalance Diet principles.

In the following section of this chapter, an extensive list of non-compliant foods and drinks will be provided. The list will include detailed information such as serving size, Glycemic Index (GI), Glycemic Load (GL), and Net Carbohydrates for each item. These metrics are particularly relevant when a food or drink item's non-compliance is attributed to a high glycemic load and/or high carbohydrate content.

Some items are deemed non-compliant due to factors like extensive processing, excessive sodium content, or high levels of unhealthy fats. For these specific items, detailed GI, GL, or net carb data may not be provided. Instead, they will be listed with a note indicating their non-compliant status, aimed at ensuring clarity in understanding why certain items are not recommended under the principles of the DiabeteBalance Diet.

▤ Banana Milkshake, 1 cup (240ml): GI of 66, GL of 39.6, Net carb= 60g

▤ Birch Beer, 1 cup (240ml): GI of 68, GL of 23.1, Net carb= 34g

▤ Bubble (Boba) Tea, 1 cup (240ml): GI of 70, GL of 42, Net carb= 60g

▤ Caramel Frappuccino, 1 cup (240ml): GI of 45, GL of 30.2, Net carb= 67g

▤ Carbonated Lemonade, 1 cup (240ml): GI of 72, GL of 21.6, Net carb= 30g

▤ Chocolate Banana Smoothie, 1 cup (240ml): GI of 45, GL of 30.6, Net carb= 68g

▤ Cola, 1 cup (240ml): GI of 63, GL of 16.4, Net carb= 26g

▤ Commercial Dairy Drinks Regular: Non-compliant foods

▤ Commercial Flavored Coffee Drinks: Non-compliant foods

▤ Commercial Frappuccino's Made: Non-compliant foods

▤ Commercial Fruit Drink Made: Non-compliant foods

▤ Commercial Fruit Juice Made: Non-compliant foods

▤ Commercial Vegetable Drink Made: Non-compliant foods

▤ Commercial Vegetables Juice Made: Non-compliant foods

▤ Cookies and Cream Milkshake, 1 cup (240ml): GI of 60, GL of 48, Net carb= 80g

▤ Cream Soda, 1 cup (240ml): GI of 71, GL of 21.3, Net carb= 30g

▤ Energy Drink (regular), 1 cup (240ml): GI of 72, GL of 20.2, Net carb= 28g

▤ Energy Drinks: Non-compliant foods

▤ Energy Shot, 1 cup (240ml): GI of 70, GL of 21, Net carb= 30g

▤ Fruit Soda, 1 cup (240ml): GI of 72, GL of 19.4, Net carb= 27g

▤ Flavored Waters with Added Sugars: Non-compliant foods

▤ Frappuccino, 1 cup (240ml): GI of 50, GL of 25, Net carb= 50g

▤ Fruit Punch, 1 cup (240ml): GI of 67, GL of 18.8, Net carb= 28g

▤ Ginger Ale, 1 cup (240ml): GI of 63, GL of 16.4, Net carb= 26g

▤ Ginger Beer, 1 cup (240ml): GI of 60, GL of 24, Net carb= 40g

▤ Grape Soda, 1 cup (240ml): GI of 63, GL of 25.2, Net carb= 40g

▤ Horchata, 1 cup (240ml): GI of 70, GL of 30.1, Net carb= 43g

▤ Hot Chocolate, 1 cup (240ml): GI of 60, GL of 18, Net carb= 30g

▤ Hot Chocolate with Whipped Cream, 1 cup (240ml): GI of 63, GL of 22.1, Net carb= 35g

▤ Hot Cider, 1 cup (240ml): GI of 65, GL of 16.9, Net carb= 26g

▤ Iced Caramel Latte, 1 cup (240ml): GI of 60, GL of 21.6, Net carb= 36g

▤ Iced Mocha, 1 cup (240ml): GI of 63, GL of 22.1, Net carb= 35g

▤ Iced Vanilla Latte, 1 cup (240ml): GI of 60, GL of 19.8, Net carb= 33g

▤ Lemon-Lime Soda, 1 cup (240ml): GI of 63, GL of 16.4, Net carb= 26g

▤ Long Island Iced Tea, 1 cup (240ml): GI of 70, GL of 30.8, Net carb= 44g

▤ Malted Milk, 1 cup (240ml): GI of 50, GL of 22.5, Net carb= 45g

▤ Milkshakes with Added Sugars: Non-compliant foods

▤ Mocha, 1 cup (240ml): GI of 55, GL of 22, Net carb= 40g

▤ Mocha Frappuccino, 1 cup (240ml): GI of 65, GL of 42.3, Net carb= 65g

▤ Red Soda, 1 cup (240ml): GI of 63, GL of 19.5, Net carb= 31g

▤ Oat Milk, sweetened, 1 cup (240ml): GI of 70, GL of 16.8, Net carb= 24g

▤ Orange carbonated drink, 1 cup (240ml): GI of 72, GL of 20.2, Net carb= 28g

▤ Orange Soda, 1 cup (240ml): GI of 63, GL of 19.5, Net carb= 31g

▤ Peach Milkshake, 1 cup (240ml): GI of 40, GL of 28, Net carb= 70g

▤ Soda with cola regular, 1 cup (240ml): GI of 63, GL of 16.4, Net carb= 26g

▤ Pina Colada, 1 cup (240ml): GI of 70, GL of 22.4, Net carb= 32g

▤ Pre-packaged Iced Tea: Non-compliant foods

▤ Pumpkin Spice Latte, 1 cup (240ml): GI of 70, GL of 36.4, Net carb= 52g

▤ Rice Milk, 1 cup (240ml): GI of 86, GL of 18.9, Net carb= 22g

▤ Rice Milk, sweetened, 1 cup (240ml): GI of 91, GL of 27.3, Net carb= 30g

▤ Root Beer, 1 cup (240ml): GI of 63, GL of 18.9, Net carb= 30g

▤ Smoothies with Added Sugars: Non-compliant foods

▤ Soda Regular : Non-compliant foods

▤ Spiced Pumpkin Latte, 1 cup (240ml): GI of 70, GL of 35, Net carb= 50g

▤ Sports Drink (regular), 1 cup (240ml): GI of 78, GL of 10.9, Net carb= 14g

▤ Sports Drinks with added sugars.: Non-compliant foods

▤ Sprite, 1 cup (240ml): GI of 63, GL of 16.4, Net carb= 26g

▤ Strawberry Milkshake, 1 cup (240ml): GI of 30, GL of 18, Net carb= 60g

▤ Sweetened Condensed Milk, 1 cup (240ml): GI of 61, GL of 101.3, Net carb= 166g

▦ Sweetened Iced Tea: Non-compliant foods

▦ Sweetened Plant-Based Milk Alternatives: Non-compliant foods

▦ Vanilla Milkshake, 1 cup (240ml): GI of 35, GL of 21, Net carb= 60g

▦ White Chocolate Mocha, 1 cup (240ml): GI of 43, GL of 25.8, Net carb= 60g

▦ White Hot Chocolate, 1 cup (240ml): GI of 50, GL of 20, Net carb= 40g

▦ Sweetened Iced Tea: Non-compliant foods

▦ Sweetened Plant-Based Milk Alternatives: Non-compliant foods

▦ Vanilla Milkshake, 1 cup (240ml): GI of 35, GL of 21, Net carb= 60g

DAIRY AND PLANT-BASED ALTERNATIVES

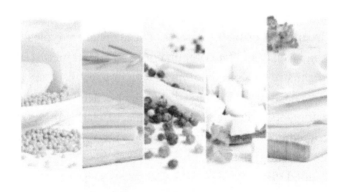

Dairy products and plant-based alternatives are often key elements of many diets due to their nutritional benefits. However, some products within this category do not adhere to the principles of the DiabeteBalance Diet.

Non-compliant items within this category typically meet at least one of several criteria. These include excessive carbohydrates, high levels of added sugars, substantial processing, unhealthy fats, high sodium levels, high glycemic load, or the inclusion of harmful preservatives that can exacerbate inflammation.

Consuming these products can negatively impact blood sugar control, overall health, and potentially contribute to inflammation-related complications. Therefore, it's important to exercise caution when incorporating dairy or plant-based alternatives into your diet.

- **Full-fat Dairy: Full-fat Dairy:** Full-fat dairy items, such as whole milk, cheese, and cream, can be rich in saturated fats, which may contribute to weight gain and cardiovascular problems.
- **Flavored Milk and Yogurts:** These often contain added sugars and artificial flavors, leading to higher carbohydrate and calorie content, making them unsuitable for the DiabeteBalance Diet.
- **Ice Cream and Frozen Desserts:** These products typically have high sugar and fat content, contributing to increased blood glucose levels and potential weight gain.
- **Processed Cheeses:** Processed cheese products can contain unhealthy fats, excessive sodium, and artificial additives that can contribute to inflammation and are inconsistent with the DiabeteBalance Diet.
- **Sweetened Plant-Based Milks:** While plant-based milks can be good alternatives to dairy, flavored or sweetened versions often contain added sugars and should be avoided.
- **Plant-Based Yogurts with Added Sugars or Artificial Additives:** Some plant-based yogurts can be high in added sugars or contain artificial additives, making them less suitable for the DiabeteBalance Diet.
- **Vegan Cheese Alternatives:** Some of these products are highly processed and can contain unhealthy fats and high

levels of sodium, which makes them non-compliant with the DiabeteBalance Diet.

For healthier choices, opt for low-fat dairy products, unsweetened plant-based milks, and plain yogurts (dairy or plant-based) without any added sugars or artificial flavors.

CHEESE AND DAIRY PRODUCTS

Dairy products and their alternatives can bring essential nutrients to a diet, but it's critical to be discerning in your choices. Some varieties can contradict the guidelines of the DiabeteBalance Diet, especially those that are processed, flavored, or have high sodium content.

Cheese varieties, such as flavored slices, processed options, or sweet cream cheese spreads, often hide additives and sugars that can trigger rapid blood glucose spikes. Their nutritional value may be compromised by processing, and high sodium content—common in some shredded cheeses and cheese dips—may undermine blood sugar management efforts. Be sure to examine labels meticulously to select options that support T2D management and overall health.

▤ American Cheese Slices ▤ Blue Cheese ▤ Cheddar Cheese Slices ▤ Cheez Whiz ▤ Colby Jack Cheese Slices ▤ Shredded Cheese ▤ String Cheese ▤ Feta Cheese ▤ Frigo Cheese Heads String Cheese ▤ Galbani String Cheese ▤ Gorgonzola Cheese ▤ Halloumi Cheese ▤ Mozzarella String Cheese ▤ Parmesan Cheese ▤ Pecorino Romano Cheese ▤ Processed Cheese ▤ Provolone Cheese Slices ▤ Roquefort Cheese ▤ Sweet Cream Cheese Spreads ▤ Vegan Cheese Alternatives

SWEETENED DAIRY PRODUCTS:

It's important to be aware of the pitfalls of sweetened dairy products. Flavored yogurts, sweetened milk, and processed cheese often contain added sugars, unhealthy fats, preservatives, and other additives. These contradict the principles of the DiabeteBalance Diet, which leans towards natural, minimally processed foods, echoing the Mediterranean Diet (MedDiet).

FULL-FAT DAIRY PRODUCTS:

While dairy can be a valuable source of protein and calcium, full-fat versions such as whole milk, cream, and full-fat cheeses can lead to excessive intake of saturated fats, conflicting with the DGA's recommendations for heart health. High-fat dairy products can also contribute to weight gain, making diabetes management more challenging.

SWEETENED PLANT-BASED MILK ALTERNATIVES:

The world of plant-based milk alternatives offers a myriad of choices, but not all are created equal. Sweetened or flavored versions often hide added sugars that can cause blood sugar levels to surge. Moreover, they might not provide the same level of essential nutrients as their unsweetened counterparts. Such products contradict the principles of the DiabeteBalance Diet, particularly the emphasis on low GL and balanced nutrient intake.

These products do not align with the GL framework and balanced nutrition principles of the DiabeteBalance Diet:

▤ Flavored almond-based yogurt drinks/smoothies ▤ Flavored coconut-based butter/margarine ▤ Flavored coconut-based coffee creamer ▤ Flavored coconut-based cream cheese ▤ Flavored coconut-based ice cream ▤ Flavored coconut-based sour cream ▤ Flavored coconut-based whipped cream ▤ Flavored coconut-based yogurt ▤ Flavored flax milk ▤ Flavored hemp milk ▤ Flavored oat milk ▤ Flavored oat-based yogurt ▤ Flavored oat-based yogurt drinks/smoothies ▤ Flavored soy-based yogurt drinks/smoothies ▤ Sweetened almond milk ▤ Sweetened almond-based butter/margarine ▤ Sweetened almond-based cheese spreads/dips ▤ Sweetened almond-based coffee creamer ▤ Sweetened almond-based cream cheese ▤ Sweetened almond-based ice cream ▤ Sweetened almond-based sour cream ▤ Sweetened almond-based whipped cream ▤ Sweetened almond-based yogurt ▤ Sweetened cashew milk ▤ Sweetened cashew-based yogurt ▤ Sweetened coconut milk ▤ Sweetened coconut-based yogurt drinks/smoothies ▤ Sweetened hazelnut milk ▤ Sweetened macadamia nut milk ▤ Sweetened oat-based butter/margarine ▤ Sweetened oat-based coffee creamer ▤ Sweetened oat-based cream cheese ▤ Sweetened oat-based sour cream ▤ Sweetened oat-based whipped cream ▤ Sweetened pea milk ▤ Sweetened rice milk ▤ Sweetened rice-based ice cream ▤ Sweetened soy milk ▤ Sweetened soy-based butter/margarine ▤ Sweetened soy-based coffee creamer ▤ Sweetened soy-based cream cheese ▤ Sweetened soy-based ice cream ▤ Sweetened soy-based sour cream ▤ Sweetened soy-based whipped cream ▤ Sweetened soy-based yogurt ▤ Sweetened walnut milk

---

HIGHLY PROCESSED PLANT-BASED ALTERNATIVES:

Many plant-based products undergo extensive processing and often contain added sugars, unhealthy fats, and elevated sodium levels. For instance, some vegan cheeses and meat substitutes fall into this category. These items do not conform to the MedDiet and 2020-2025 Dietary Guidelines for Americans for low sodium intake, minimally processed foods, and balanced nutrient intake:

▦ Plant-based butter ▦ Plant-based cheese blocks/wheels ▦ Plant-based cheese dips/spreads ▦ Plant-based cheese sauces ▦ Plant-based cheese slices ▦ Plant-based cheese spreads/dips ▦ Plant-based cheese-filled breadsticks ▦ Plant-based cheese-filled pasta (e.g., vegan stuffed shells, vegan ravioli) ▦ Plant-based cheese-filled pastries (e.g., vegan cheese danishes, vegan cheese croissants) ▦ Plant-based cheese-filled pretzels ▦ Plant-based cheese-filled quesadillas ▦ Plant-based cheese-filled sandwiches/burgers ▦ Plant-based cheese-filled snacks (e.g., vegan cheese puffs, vegan cheese balls) ▦ Plant-based cheese-filled tarts ▦ Plant-based cheese-filled wraps/burritos ▦ Plant-based cheese-flavored biscuits ▦ Plant-based cheese-flavored bread ▦ Plant-based cheese-flavored breaded products (e.g., vegan cheese sticks, vegan cheese bites) ▦ Plant-based cheese-flavored crackers ▦ Plant-based cheese-flavored crackers/chips ▦ Plant-based cheese-flavored crackers/crisps ▦ Plant-based cheese-flavored dips for chips/crackers ▦ Plant-based cheese-flavored dips for vegetables/crackers ▦ Plant-based cheese-flavored dressings for salads ▦ Plant-based cheese-flavored dressings for sandwiches/wraps ▦ Plant-based cheese-flavored frozen appetizers (e.g., vegan cheese sticks, vegan cheese bites) ▦ Plant-based cheese-flavored instant meals ▦ Plant-based cheese-flavored popcorn ▦ Plant-based cheese-flavored popcorn seasoning ▦ Plant-based cheese-flavored protein bars ▦ Plant-based cheese-flavored puffs/corn snacks ▦ Plant-based cheese-flavored rice cakes ▦ Plant-based cheese-flavored rice/pasta dishes ▦ Plant-based cheese-flavored salad dressings ▦ Plant-based cheese-flavored sauces for nachos ▦ Plant-based cheese-flavored sauces for pasta ▦ Plant-based cheese-flavored seasoning mixes ▦ Plant-based cheese-flavored seasonings for popcorn/fries ▦ Plant-based cheese-flavored snack bars ▦ Plant-based cheese-flavored vegetable chips ▦ Plant-based cheese-flavored vegetable spreads ▦ Plant-based cheese-stuffed crusts (e.g., vegan stuffed crust pizza) ▦ Plant-based chocolate milk ▦ Plant-based coffee creamers ▦ Plant-based condensed milk ▦ Plant-based cream cheese ▦ Plant-based cream-filled pastries (e.g., sweetened vegan cream puffs) ▦ Plant-based creamer for cooking/baking ▦ Plant-based creamer for desserts ▦ Plant-based creamer for soups/sauces ▤ Plant-based creamers for tea/hot beverages ▤ Plant-based custards/puddings ▤ Plant-based frozen yogurt ▤ Plant-based half-and-half ▤ Plant-based ice cream ▤ Plant-based margarine ▤ Plant-based milkshakes ▤ Plant-based smoothies ▤ Plant-based sour cream ▤ Plant-based whipped cream ▤ Plant-based whipped toppings ▤ Plant-based whipped toppings for desserts ▤ Plant-based yogurt drinks ▤ Vegan cheddar shreds (with preservatives or additives) ▤ Vegan cheese bites (with preservatives or additives) ▤ Vegan cheese sticks (with preservatives or additives) ▤ Vegan mozzarella shreds (with preservatives or additives)

Instead, opt for unsweetened, low-fat, or non-fat dairy products and unsweetened, fortified plant-based alternatives. These options align better with the principles of a healthy, balanced diet, as they offer essential nutrients without the adverse effects of high sugar, unhealthy fats, and high sodium content.

OTHER DAIRY AND ALTERNATIVES WITH HIGH CARB AND/OR HIGH SODIUM CONTENT

▤ Banoffee Pie ▤ Brigadeiro ▤ Coconut Ice ▤ Coconut Macadamia Balls ▤ Coconut Macaroons ▤ Dessert-Style Plant-Based Puddings ▤ Easy Cheese ▤ Flan/Caramel Custard ▤ Flavored Milk ▤ Flavored Plant-Based Yogurts ▤ Flavored Soy Milk ▤ Flavored Yogurt ▤ Fritos Jalapeno Cheddar Cheese Dip ▤ Fruit Yogurt Parfaits ▤ Fudge Brownies ▤ Fudge ▤ Ice Cream ▤ Icebox Cake ▤ Key Lime Pie ▤ Lemon Bars ▤ Magic Bars ▤ Instant Macaroni and Cheese ▤ Milkshakes ▤ Nacho Cheese Sauce ▤ Plant-Based Creamers ▤ Plant-Based Dessert Alternatives ▤ Gourmet Nacho Cheese Sauce ▤ Sweetened Almond Milk ▤ Sweetened Cashew Milk ▤ Sweetened Coconut Milk ▤ Sweetened Condensed Milk ▤ Sweetened Oat Milk ▤ Sweetened Plant-Based Creamers ▤ Sweetened Rice Milk ▤ Sweetened Whipped Cream ▤ Tres Leches Cake ▤ Vietnamese Coffee

DIPS AND DRESSINGS

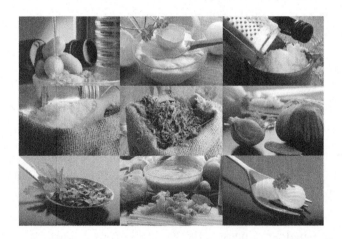

As an individual navigating Type 2 Diabetes (T2D), the choice of dips and dressings can significantly impact the adherence to the Diabete-Balance Diet. While they might seem like minor components of a meal, dips and dressings can, in fact, carry a substantial nutritional load that affects blood glucose control and overall health.

The DiabeteBalance Diet places emphasis on natural, minimally processed foods, controlled sodium and sugar intake, and healthy fats, among other factors.

However, not all dips and dressings align with these principles. Some may be laden with added sugars, packed with excessive sodium, harbor unhealthy fats, or contain artificial additives. Consumption of such products can impede blood sugar control, compromise overall health, and hamper effective T2D management.

The subsequent sections of this chapter will delve into specific categories of dips and dressings that are non-compliant with the Diabete-Balance Diet and explain the reasons for their non-compliance. The aim is to guide you in making informed decisions when selecting dips and dressings that align with their dietary goals and support the effective management of diabetes.

CREAMY AND FULL-FAT DRESSINGS

Dressings such as ranch, blue cheese, and thousand island are commonly known for their high levels of saturated fats and calories. Consuming these dressings in excess can potentially lead to weight gain and elevated blood glucose levels. Dressings that do not align with the low GL, reduced calorie, and low saturated fat principles of the DiabeteBalance Diet include:

▤ Avocado ranch dressing ▤ Blue cheese dressing ▤ Buttermilk dressing ▤ Caesar dressing ▤ Chipotle ranch dressing ▤ Creamy almond dressing ▤ Creamy avocado dressing ▤ Creamy bacon dressing ▤ Creamy balsamic dressing ▤ Creamy blue cheese dressing ▤ Creamy Caesar dressing ▤ Creamy cashew dressing ▤ Creamy chipotle dressing ▤ Creamy cilantro lime dressing ▤ Creamy coconut dressing ▤ Creamy cucumber dressing ▤ Creamy curry dressing ▤ Creamy dill dressing ▤ Creamy French dressing ▤ Creamy garlic dressing ▤ Creamy ginger dressing ▤ Creamy ginger miso dressing ▤ Creamy honey mustard dressing ▤ Creamy horseradish dressing ▤ Creamy Italian dressing ▤ Creamy Italian herb dressing ▤ Creamy lemon herb dressing ▤ Creamy macadamia nut dressing ▤ Creamy mango dressing ▤ Creamy maple dijon dressing ▤ Creamy Parmesan dressing ▤ Creamy peanut dressing ▤ Creamy pecan dressing ▤ Creamy pesto dressing ▤ Creamy pineapple dressing ▤ Creamy ranch dressing ▤ Creamy roasted garlic dressing ▤ Creamy Russian dressing ▤ Creamy sesame dressing ▤ Creamy sesame ginger dressing ▤ Creamy sriracha dressing ▤ Creamy sun-dried tomato dressing ▤ Creamy sunflower seed dressing ▤ Creamy sweet chili dressing ▤ Creamy tahini dressing ▤ Creamy walnut dressing ▤ Green goddess dressing ▤ Honey mustard dressing (creamy variety) ▤ Ranch dressing ▤ Thousand Island dressing

SUGARY DRESSINGS:

Some dressings, including certain types of vinaigrettes and sweet dressings like honey mustard, can be high in added sugars. Consuming these dressings can result in rapid blood sugar spikes, which is a factor of non-compliance with the GL framework of the DiabeteBalance Diet.

▤ Apricot vinaigrette ▤ Asian sesame dressing ▤ Balsamic glaze ▤ Banana dressing ▤ Blackberry vinaigrette ▤ Blueberry dressing ▤ Brown sugar bacon dressing ▤ Brown sugar bourbon dressing ▤ Brown sugar dressing ▤ Candied pecan dressing ▤ Caramelized onion dressing ▤ Cherry vinaigrette ▤ Cinnamon honey dressing ▤ Coconut lime dressing ▤ Cranberry vinaigrette ▤ Creamy blue cheese dressing with sweet additions ▤ Creamy candied bacon dressing ▤ Creamy caramel apple dressing ▤ Creamy caramelized onion dressing ▤ Creamy coconut lime dressing ▤ Creamy fruit dressing ▤ Creamy honey balsamic dressing ▤ Creamy honey chipotle dressing ▤ Creamy honey lime dressing ▤ Creamy honey mustard dressing ▤ Creamy honey sesame dressing ▤ Creamy honey sriracha dressing ▤ Creamy pecan praline dressing ▤ Creamy raspberry walnut dressing ▤ Fig balsamic dressing ▤ French dressing ▤ Grape dressing ▤ Grapefruit vinaigrette ▤ Hibiscus dressing ▤ Honey almond dressing ▤ Honey mustard dressing ▤ Key lime dressing ▤ Lemon poppy seed dressing ▤ Lemonade dressing ▤ Mango vinaigrette ▤ Maple bacon vinaigrette ▤ Maple pecan vinaigrette ▤ Maple vinaigrette ▤ Orange ginger dressing ▤ Peach vinaigrette ▤ Pineapple dressing ▤ Pomegranate dressing ▤ Poppy seed dressing ▤ Raspberry chipotle dressing ▤ Raspberry vinaigrette ▤ Strawberry dressing ▤ Sweet and creamy avocado lime dressing ▤ Sweet and creamy bacon ranch dressing ▤ Sweet and creamy pecan maple dressing ▤ Sweet and creamy poppy seed dressing ▤ Sweet and creamy sesame ginger dressing ▤ Sweet and sour dressing ▤ Sweet and tangy ranch dressing ▤ Sweet chili sauce ▤ Sweet onion dressing ▤ Teriyaki glaze ▤ Thousand Island dressing ▤ Vanilla bean dressing ▤ Watermelon vinaigrette

PROCESSED DIPS (COMMERCIALLY MADE)

Many commercially available dips, such as some varieties of salsa, queso, and spinach dip, can be heavily processed and high in sodium. They may also contain added sugars and/or unhealthy fats. The high sodium content and the processed nature of these dips make them incompatible with the MedDiet and DGA's emphasis on lower sodium and minimally processed foods. These products include:

▤ Artichoke and parmesan dip ▤ Artichoke and spinach dip ▤ Bacon and cheddar dip ▤ Bacon ranch dip ▤ Barbecue bacon dip ▤ BBQ ranch dip ▤ Black bean dip ▤ Buffalo cauliflower dip ▤ Buffalo chicken dip ▤ Buffalo ranch dip ▤ Caramel apple dip ▤ Caramelized onion dip ▤ Cheeseburger dip ▤ Cheesy spinach dip ▤ Chili cheese dip ▤ Chipotle bacon dip ▤ Chocolate chip cookie dough dip ▤

Cilantro lime dip ▦ Crab dip ▦ Crab Rangoon dip ▦ Creamy dill dip ▦ Cucumber and dill dip ▦ Dill pickle dip ▦ Fiesta cheese dip ▦ French onion dip ▦ Greek tzatziki dip ▦ Honey mustard dip ▦ Honey sriracha dip ▦ Horseradish dip ▦ Hot bacon dip ▦ Jalapeno cheese dip ▦ Jalapeno popper dip ▦ Lemon herb dip ▦ Loaded baked potato dip ▦ Loaded nacho dip ▦ Mango salsa dip ▦ Olive tapenade dip ▦ Pepperoni pizza dip ▦ Pimento cheese dip ▦ Queso dip ▦ Ranch dip ▦ Roasted eggplant dip ▦ Roasted garlic dip ▦ Roasted red pepper dip ▦ S'mores dip ▦ Salsa con queso dip ▦ Seven-layer dip ▦ Smoked salmon dip ▦ Smoky chipotle dip ▦ Sour cream and onion dip ▦ Southwest fiesta dip ▦ Spicy avocado dip ▦ Spicy buffalo dip ▦ Spinach and artichoke dip ▦ Sriracha dip ▦ Sun-dried tomato dip ▦ Sweet and spicy mustard dip ▦ Sweet chili dip ▦ Tomato and basil dip ▦ White bean dip

---

CHEESE-BASED DIPS

While delicious, these dips often contain high amounts of saturated fats, added sugar, and calories. They typically do not align with the principles of balanced nutrient intake and reduced saturated fat content inherent to the DiabeteBalance Diet.

▦ Asiago and roasted garlic dip ▦ Asiago and sun-dried tomato dip ▦ Bacon and cheddar dip ▦ Beer cheese dip ▦ Blue cheese and bacon dip ▦ Blue cheese and walnut dip ▦ Blue cheese dip ▦ Boursin cheese dip ▦ Brie and cranberry dip ▦ Brie and honey dip ▦ Buffalo chicken dip ▦ Camembert and cranberry dip ▦ Camembert and fig dip ▦ Cheddar and beer dip ▦ Cheddar and green onion dip ▦ Cheesy bacon dip ▦ Cheesy buffalo dip ▦ Chili cheese dip ▦ Chipotle cheese dip ▦ Colby and horseradish dip ▦ Colby Jack dip ▦ Creamy feta dip ▦ Edam and chive dip ▦ Feta and roasted red pepper dip ▦ Feta and spinach dip ▦ Fontina and mushroom dip ▦ Fontina and roasted pepper dip ▦ Fontina and spinach dip ▦ Four cheese dip ▦ Garlic and herb cheese dip ▦ Goat cheese and apricot dip ▦ Gorgonzola and caramelized onion dip ▦ Gorgonzola dip ▦ Gouda and caramelized onion dip ▦ Gruyere and bacon dip ▦ Gruyere and caramelized onion dip ▦ Havarti and dill dip ▦ Havarti and sun-dried tomato dip ▦ Havarti and sun-dried tomato dip ▦ Horseradish cheddar dip ▦ Jalapeno popper dip ▦ Mexican queso dip ▦ Monterey Jack and jalapeno dip ▦ Monterey Jack dip ▦ Mozzarella and basil dip ▦ Mozzarella and pesto dip ▦ Parmesan and artichoke dip ▦ Parmesan and black pepper dip ▦ Pepper Jack and bacon dip ▦ Pepper Jack and habanero dip ▦ Pepper Jack and jalapeno dip ▦ Pepper Jack dip ▦ Pimento cheese dip ▦ Provolone and Italian herbs dip ▦ Provolone and roasted red pepper dip ▦ Queso dip ▦ Ranch dip ▦ Ricotta and herb dip ▦ Ricotta and roasted garlic dip ▦ Roquefort and walnut dip ▦ Roquefort dip ▦ Smoked cheddar dip ▦ Smoked Gouda and bacon dip ▦ Smoked Gouda and chipotle dip ▦ Smoked Gouda dip ▦ Spinach and cheese dip ▦ Stilton and walnut dip ▦ Swiss and caramelized onion dip ▦ Swiss and mushroom dip ▦ Swiss cheese dip

Instead of these non-compliant options, opt for healthier dips and dressings. Consider homemade vinaigrettes made with olive oil, vinegar, and herbs, or dips made from Greek yogurt or mashed avocado. Hummus can also be a healthy option. These choices can offer the flavor and texture you seek without the negative impacts on your blood sugar and overall health. As always, moderation is key even with healthier choices.

GRAINS, CEREALS AND PASTA

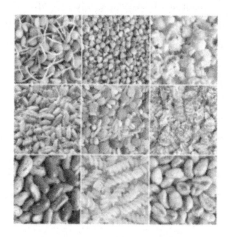

As foundations of many traditional diets, grains, cereals, and pasta have a prominent place on our tables. However, when managing diabetes, it is essential to scrutinize these carbohydrate-rich staples closely. While these foods provide energy, they can also impact blood glucose levels due to their varying glycemic index (GI), glycemic load (GL), and nutrient composition. Therefore, certain categories of these foods may be incompatible with the principles of the DiabeteBalance Diet.

- **Refined Grains:** Refined grains, including white bread, white rice, and conventional pasta, undergo extensive processing that removes the fiber and nutrient-rich outer layers. This refining process results in easily digestible carbohydrates that quickly raise blood glucose levels after consumption. For individuals aiming to control or reverse T2D, these refined grains are not an option.

- **Sugary Cereals:** Many breakfast cereals available in supermarkets are loaded with added sugars, making them unsuitable for the DiabeteBalance Diet. These cereals often lack sufficient fiber and protein content to slow down digestion and prevent rapid blood sugar spikes. Therefore, it is important to carefully read product labels, select cereals with minimal added sugars, and explore healthier breakfast alternatives.

- **Flavored Instant Oatmeal:** While flavored instant oatmeal may appear convenient and delicious, they often contain excessive amounts of added sugars and artificial flavorings. These additives undermine the nutritional value of the oats. Opting for plain oats or steel-cut oats, which are minimally processed, and sweetening them naturally with spices or fruits is a healthier choice.

- **Pasta made from Refined Grains:** Pasta made from refined wheat flour poses similar challenges as other refined grains, as it is quickly digested and can lead to significant blood sugar increases. Instead, choosing whole grain or whole wheat pasta, which is higher in fiber and nutrients, is a better option for those seeking to reverse T2D.

- **Pre-packaged Rice Mixes:** Pre-packaged rice mixes often contain high levels of sodium, artificial flavorings, and unnecessary additives, which can be detrimental for individuals managing T2D. These mixes not only contribute to high blood pressure but may also contain hidden sugars. Preparing brown rice or quinoa at home allows for better control over the ingredients and aligns with a healthier the DiabeteBalance Diet.

In the following section of this chapter, an expanded list of non-compliant foods within the DiabeteBalance Diet is provided. Each food item is accompanied by detailed information, including serving size, Glycemic Index (GI), Glycemic Load (GL), and Net Carbohydrates. Some foods, due to reasons such as extensive processing or high sodium content, may not have detailed GI, GL, or net carb data. Instead, their non-compliant status is clearly indicated, offering a comprehensive understanding of why certain foods are not suitable within the DiabeteBalance Diet.

▤ Barley Flour or Meal, ½ cup, 64g: GI of 55, , GL of 12, Net carb= 38g

▤ Barley Malt Flour, ½ cup, 61g: GI of 65, , GL of 18, Net carb= 42g

▤ Calrose Rice, ½ cup cooked, 80g: GI of 75, , GL of 27.5, Net carb= 37g

▤ Canned Pasta Meals: Non-compliant foods

▤ Cereal Bars (different brands) : Non-compliant foods

▤ Cinnamon Toast Crunch, 1 cup, 31g: GI of 74, , GL of 16, Net carb= 24g

▤ Cinnamon Toast Crunch: Non-compliant foods

▤ Chocolate Chunks (different brands), 1 cup, 27g: GI of 77, , GL of 23, Net carb= 24g

▤ Corn Flakes (different brands), 1 cup, 28g: GI of 93, , GL of 18, Net carb= 23g

▤ Corn Flour Masa White, 1 cup, 114g: GI of 60-65, , GL of 42, Net carb= 77g

▤ Corn Flour Whole-Grain Blue, 1 cup, 128g: GI of 50-55, , GL of 34, Net carb= 76g

▤ Corn Flour Whole-Grain White, 1 cup, 128g: GI of 50-55, , GL of 34, Net carb= 76g

▤ Corn Flour Whole-Grain Yellow, 1 cup, 128g: GI of 50-55, , GL of 34, Net carb= 76g

▤ Corn Flour Yellow Degermed, 1 cup, 125g: GI of 50-55, , GL of 31, Net carb= 71g

▤ Corn Pops (different brands): Non-compliant foods

▤ Cornmeal Degermed White, 1 cup, 138g: GI of 50-55, , GL of 32, Net carb= 75g

▤ Cornmeal Degermed White, 1 cup, 138g: GI of 50-55, , GL of 32, Net carb= 75g

▤ Cornmeal Degermed Yellow, 1 cup, 138g: GI of 50-55, , GL of 32, Net carb= 75g

▤ Cornstarch, 1 cup, 128g: GI of 85-90, , GL of 43, Net carb= 107g

▤ Count Chocula: Non-compliant foods

▤ Cream of Rice (different brands), 1 cup cooked, 240g: GI of 70-85, , GL of 20, Net carb= 27g

▤ Cream of Wheat (different brands), 1 cup cooked, 244g: GI of 70-85, , GL of 19, Net carb= 26g

▤ Farina, 1 cup cooked, 242g: GI of 70-80, , GL of 19, Net carb= 26g

▤ Farro, 1 cup cooked, 169g: GI of 40, , GL of 18, Net carb= 45g

▤ Glazed Sugar Flakes types (different brands), 1 cup, 27g: GI of 55, , GL of 16, Net carb= 26g

▤ Garlic and Herb Penne, 2 ounces, 56g: GI of 50, , GL of 18, Net carb= 41g

▤ Gluten Free Corn Noodles, 1 cup, 200g: GI of 60-65, , GL of 27, Net carb= 42g

▤ Gluten-Free Penne, 2 ounces, 56g: GI of 40, , GL of 10, Net carb= 43g

▤ Gluten-Free Spaghetti, 1 cup cooked, 140g: GI of 52, , GL of 24, Net carb= 46g

▤ Glutinous Rice, 1 cup cooked, 174g: GI of 86-91, , GL of 37, Net carb= 42g

▤ Granola, 1/2 cup, 61g: GI of 56-69, , GL of 17, Net carb= 37g

▤ Instant Flavored Rice or Pasta Mixes: Non-compliant foods

▤ Instant Oatmeal Packs (different brands) : Non-compliant foods

▤ Muesli with Added Sugars (different brands) : Non-compliant foods

▤ Pop-Tarts Cereal: Non-compliant foods

▤ Processed Bran Cereals (different brands) : Non-compliant foods

▤ Puffed Rice or Corn Cereals (different brands) : Non-compliant foods

▤ Seasoned Packaged Noodles: Non-compliant foods

▤ Sugar-Sweetened Flakes (different brands) : Non-compliant foods

▤ Sugary Cereals (different brands) : Non-compliant foods

FISH, SEAFOOD, AND FISH PRODUCTS

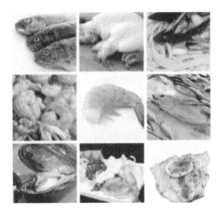

While fish and seafood are generally considered beneficial for the DiabeteBalance Diet due to their lean protein content, omega-3 fatty acids, and low glycemic load (GL), it's essential to be aware of specific variations that may not align with this dietary approach.

Some preparations or processing methods can result in high sodium content, extensive processing, breading, and certain cooking methods that can potentially undermine the health benefits of fish and seafood for individuals managing T2D and aiming for weight loss, as per the twins cycle hypothesis.

These factors can transform what are typically healthy options into choices that may not be conducive to blood sugar control and overall health in the context of T2D management. It is crucial to be selective in choosing fish and seafood preparations that prioritize minimal processing, low sodium content, and healthier cooking methods such as grilling or baking.

Here are some categories that do not comply with the diet's principles:

- **Breaded and Fried Fish:** Although fish is naturally low in unhealthy fats and carbohydrates, when it's breaded and fried, it becomes a less healthy option. The breading, often composed of refined grains, introduces additional carbohydrates that can elevate blood sugar levels. Frying, on the other hand, can significantly increase calorie content and potentially foster insulin resistance. Therefore, it's better to avoid breaded and fried fish on the DiabeteBalance Diet.
- **Processed Seafood Products:** Items such as fish sticks, fish patties, and seafood nuggets often involve heavy processing and may contain additives, preservatives, and unhealthy fats. High in sodium, unhealthy oils, and even hidden sugars, these processed foods are not a smart choice for T2D management. Fresh or minimally processed seafood is a far healthier alternative.
- **Smoked and Cured Fish:** Smoked and cured fish products like smoked salmon or salted fish can have a high sodium content, which is problematic for individuals with T2D. Excessive sodium intake contribute to high blood pressure and increased cardiovascular risk. Consumption of these types of fish should be minimized, and lower-sodium alternatives should be considered instead.
- **Breaded and Fried Seafood:** Just like breaded and fried fish,

breaded and fried seafood (such as shrimp or calamari) is high in unhealthy fats, calories, and refined grains. The breading and frying process can lead to blood sugar spikes and should be avoided on the DiabeteBalance Diet.

- **High Sodium Canned Fish:** Canned fish products, particularly those packed in brine or sauces, often contain excessive sodium, which can cause fluid retention and elevated blood pressure. Choosing low-sodium or no-salt-added canned fish options can help minimize these negative effects.

Although fish and seafood provide numerous health benefits, it's crucial to make informed choices for a successful the DiabeteBalance Diet. Avoid breaded and fried fish or seafood, heavily processed seafood products, smoked and cured fish, and high-sodium canned fish. Instead, prioritize fresh or minimally processed fish and seafood, and be mindful of cooking methods that minimize the addition of unhealthy fats, refined grains, and excessive sodium.

FRUITS AND FRUITS PRODUCTS

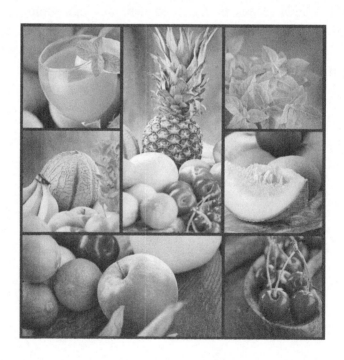

Fruit is generally regarded as a healthy and nutritious component of a balanced diet, providing essential vitamins, minerals, and fiber. However, in the context of the DiabeteBalance Diet, there are categories of fruit and fruit products that may not comply with its principles.

- **Fruit products with added sugars, fats, and sodium**: Certain fruit-based products, such as fruit snacks, canned fruits in syrup, or fruit desserts, often have added sugars, unhealthy fats, and elevated sodium levels. These additions can contribute to higher calorie content and negatively impact blood sugar control.
- **Fruit juices:** Fruit juices can have a higher glycemic index (GI) and glycemic load (GL) compared to whole fruits. They are often processed, which can lead to reduced fiber content and a quicker release of sugars into the bloodstream, potentially affecting blood sugar levels.
- **Dried fruits:** Drying fruits can lead to a concentration of sugars and a reduction in fiber content. This results in a higher glycemic impact compared to whole fruits. It is important to consume dried fruits in moderation and be mindful of portion sizes.
- **Fruit products with preservatives and artificial additives:** Some fruit products, such as canned fruits with preservatives or fruit snacks with artificial additives, may not be in line with the principles of the DiabeteBalance Diet. These additives can have negative effects on blood sugar control and overall health.

It is recommended to prioritize whole fruits and limit or avoid fruit products that fall into these non-compliant categories. By choosing whole fruits, individuals can benefit from their natural fiber content and lower glycemic impact, supporting stable blood sugar control and the goals of the DiabeteBalance Diet.

In the subsequent section of this chapter, a comprehensive list is

315

provided to outline foods that do not comply with the DiabeteBalance Diet. This list offers detailed information, including serving size, Glycemic Index (GI), Glycemic Load (GL), and Net Carbohydrates for each food item. These metrics are particularly relevant when a food item's non-compliance is attributed to its high glycemic load and/or high carbohydrate content.

▤ Apple Candied, 1 medium (60g): GI= High, GL=High, Net carb= Varies

▤ Apple Fried: Non-compliant foods

▤ Apple Jelly (store bought), 1 tbsp (20g): GI= High, GL=High, Net carb= Varies

▤ Apple Rings Fried: Non-compliant foods

▤ Apples (like in fried apple pies): Non-compliant foods

▤ Applesauce Canned Heavy Syrup Drained, 1 tbsp (20g): GI= High, GL=High, Net carb= Varies

▤ Applesauce Canned Sweetened, 1 cup (250g): GI= High, GL=High, Net carb= 43g

▤ Apricot Dried Cooked With Sugar, 1 cup (225g): GI= High, GL=High, Net carb= 51g

▤ Apricot Preserves (store bought), 1 tbsp (20g): GI= High, GL=High, Net carb= Varies

▤ Apricots Canned Heavy Syrup Drained, 1 cup (235g): GI= High, GL=High, Net carb= 38g

▤ Apricots Canned Heavy Syrup Drained, 1 tbsp (20g): GI= High, GL=High, Net carb= Varies

▤ Apricots Dehydrated Sulfured Stewed, 1 cup (245g): GI= High, GL=High, Net carb= 36g

▤ Banana Batter-Dipped Fried, 1 extra small (105g): GI= High,

GL=High, Net carb= 35g

▤ Banana Red Fried, 1 extra small (105g): GI= High, GL=High, Net carb= 35g

▤ Banana Ripe Fried, 1 extra small (105g): GI= High, GL=High, Net carb= 35g

▤ Banana, ripe, 1 extra small (105g): GI= 85, GL=26.5, Net carb= 31g

▤ Banana, ripe Baked, 1 extra small (105g): GI= High, GL=High, Net carb= 28g

▤ Bananas fritters : Non-compliant foods

▤ Blackberries Canned Heavy Syrup Drained, 1 cup (250g): GI= High, GL=High, Net carb= 36g

▤ Blackberries Canned Heavy Syrup Drained, 1 tbsp (20g): GI= High, GL=High, Net carb= Varies

▤ Blackberry Jam (store bought), 1 tbsp (20g): GI= High, GL=High, Net carb= Varies

▤ Blueberries Canned Heavy Syrup, 1 cup (256g): GI= High, GL=High, Net carb= 33g

▤ Blueberries Canned Heavy Syrup Drained, 1 tbsp (20g): GI= High, GL=High, Net carb= Varies

▤ Blueberry Jam (store bought), 1 tbsp (20g): GI= High, GL=High, Net carb= Varies

▤ Boysenberries Canned Heavy Syrup, 1 cup (250g): GI= High, GL=High, Net carb= 36g

▤ Boysenberries Canned Heavy Syrup Drained, 1 tbsp (20g): GI= High, GL=High, Net carb= Varies

▤ Cherry Jam (store bought), 1 tbsp (20g): GI= High, GL=High, Net carb= Varies

▤ Cranberry Jelly (store bought), 1 tbsp (20g): GI= High, GL=High, Net carb= Varies

▤ Cranberry sauce Canned Heavy Syrup Drained, 1 tbsp (20g): GI= High, GL=High, Net carb= Varies

▤ Cranberry sauce, Canned Heavy Syrup Drained, ¼ cup (70g): GI= High, GL=High, Net carb= Varies

▤ Dried Apricots, sweetened, ¼ cup (32g): GI= High, GL=High, Net carb= Varies

▤ Dried Banana, sweetened, ¼ cup (30g): GI= High, GL=High, Net carb= Varies

▤ Dried Blueberries, sweetened, ¼ cup (40g): GI= High, GL=High, Net carb= Varies

▤ Dried Cherries, sweetened, ¼ cup (40g): GI= High, GL=High, Net carb= Varies

▤ Dried Cranberries, sweetened, ¼ cup (40g): GI= High, GL=High, Net carb= Varies

▤ Dried Currants, sweetened, ¼ cup (40g): GI= High, GL=High, Net carb= Varies

▤ Dried Custard Apple Sweetened, ¼ cup (30g): GI= High, GL=High, Net carb= Varies

▤ Dried Kiwi, sweetened, ¼ cup (30g): GI= High, GL=High, Net carb= Varies

▤ Dried Longan, ¼ cup (32g): GI= High, GL=High, Net carb= Varies

▤ Dried Lychee, sweetened, ¼ cup (30g): GI= High, GL=High, Net carb= Varies

▤ Dried Mango, sweetened, ¼ cup (30g): GI= High, GL=High, Net carb= Varies

▤ Dried Papaya, sweetened, ¼ cup (30g): GI= High, GL=High, Net carb= Varies

▤ Dried Pear, sweetened, ¼ cup (40g): GI= High, GL=High, Net carb= Varies

▤ Dried Persimmon, ¼ cup (32g): GI= High, GL=High, Net carb= Varies

▤ Dried Persimmon, sweetened, ¼ cup (32g): GI= High, GL=High, Net carb= Varies

▤ Dried Pineapple Sweetened, ¼ cup (40g): GI= High, GL=High, Net carb= Varies

▤ Dried Pineapple, sweetened, ¼ cup (35g): GI= High, GL=High, Net carb= Varies

▤ Dried Sapodilla Sweetened, ¼ cup (30g): GI= High, GL=High, Net carb= Varies

▤ Fig Jam (store bought), 1 tbsp (20g): GI= High, GL=High, Net carb= Varies

▤ Fried Apples: Non-compliant foods

▤ Fried Mango: Non-compliant foods

▤ Fried Peaches: Non-compliant foods

▤ Fried pineapple fritters: Non-compliant foods

▤ Fried Strawberries: Non-compliant foods

▤ Golden Seedless Raisins, ¼ cup (40g): GI= High, GL=High, Net carb= Varies

▤ Grape Jelly (store bought), 1 tbsp (20g): GI= High, GL=High, Net carb= Varies

▤ Grape Juice (store bought), 1 cup (253g): GI= High, GL=High, Net carb= Varies

▤ Guava Nectar Canned, 1 cup (240g): GI= High, GL=High, Net carb= Varies

▤ Guava Nectar Canned Heavy Syrup Drained, 1 tbsp (20g): GI= High, GL=High, Net carb= Varies

▤ Kiwi Jam (store bought), 1 tbsp (20g): GI= High, GL=High, Net carb= Varies

▤ Lemon Curd (store bought), 1 tbsp (20g): GI= High, GL=High, Net carb= Varies

▤ Mango Jam (store bought), 1 tbsp (20g): GI= High, GL=High, Net carb= Varies

▤ Mango Nectar Canned Heavy Syrup Drained, 1 tbsp (20g): GI= High, GL=High, Net carb= Varies

▤ Mixed Fruit Preserves (store bought), 1 tbsp (20g): GI= High, GL=High, Net carb= Varies

▤ Nance Canned Heavy Syrup Drained, 1 cup (160g): GI= High, GL=High, Net carb= Varies

▤ Nance Canned Heavy Syrup Drained, 1 tbsp (20g): GI= High, GL=High, Net carb= Varies

▤ Orange Marmalade (store bought), 1 tbsp (20g): GI= High, GL=High, Net carb= Varies

▤ Orange Pineapple Juice Blend (store bought), 1 cup (250g): GI= High, GL=High, Net carb= Varies

▤ Peach Preserves (store bought), 1 tbsp (20g): GI= High, GL=High, Net carb= Varies

▤ Peaches Spiced Canned Heavy Syrup, 1 cup (250g): GI= High, GL=High, Net carb= Varies

▤ Peaches Spiced Canned Heavy Syrup, 1 tbsp (20g): GI= High, GL=High, Net carb= Varies

▤ Pear Preserves (store bought), 1 tbsp (20g): GI= High, GL=High, Net carb= Varies

▤ Pears Canned Heavy Syrup, 1 cup (245g): GI= High, GL=High, Net carb= Varies

▤ Pears Canned Heavy Syrup Drained, 1 cup (242g): GI= High, GL=High, Net carb= Varies

▤ Pears Canned Heavy Syrup Drained, 1 tbsp (20g): GI= High, GL=High, Net carb= Varies

▤ Pears Canned Heavy Syrup Drained, 1 tbsp (20g): GI= High, GL=High, Net carb= Varies

▤ Pineapple Canned Extra Heavy Syrup, 1 cup (250g): GI= High, GL=High, Net carb= Varies

▤ Pineapple Canned Extra Heavy Syrup, 1 tbsp (20g): GI= High, GL=High, Net carb= Varies

▤ Pineapple Canned Heavy Syrup, 1 tbsp (20g): GI= High, GL=High, Net carb= Varies

▤ Pineapple Canned Heavy Syrup Drained, 1 cup (246g): GI= High, GL=High, Net carb= Varies

▤ Pineapple Canned Heavy Syrup Drained, 1 cup (248g): GI= High, GL=High, Net carb= Varies

▤ Pineapple Canned Heavy Syrup Drained, 1 tbsp (20g): GI= High, GL=High, Net carb= Varies

▤ Pineapple Canned Heavy Syrup Drained, 1 tbsp (20g): GI= High, GL=High, Net carb= Varies

▤ Pineapple Frozen Chunks Sweetened, 1 cup (165g): GI= 58, GL=24.3, Net carb= 42g

▤ Pineapple Jam (store bought), 1 tbsp (20g): GI= High, GL=High, Net carb= Varies

◼ Pineapple, Canned Heavy Syrup Drained, ½ cup (122g): GI= High, GL=High, Net carb= Varies

◼ Plantains Cooked, ½ cup mashed (100g): GI= 55, GL=17.6, Net carb= 32g

◼ Plantains fried : Non-compliant foods

◼ Plantains Green Fried: Non-compliant foods

◼ Plum Jam (store bought), 1 tbsp (20g): GI= High, GL=High, Net carb= Varies

◼ Plums Canned Heavy Syrup Drained, ½ cup (125g): GI= High, GL=High, Net carb= Varies

◼ Plums Canned Heavy Syrup Drained, 1 tbsp (20g): GI= High, GL=High, Net carb= Varies

◼ Raisin, ¼ cup (40g): GI= 66, GL=20.5, Net carb= 31g

◼ Raspberry Jam (store bought), 1 tbsp (20g): GI= High, GL=High, Net carb= Varies

◼ Strawberry Jam (store bought), 1 tbsp (20g): GI= High, GL=High, Net carb= Varies

◼ Sweetened Dried Apples, ¼ cup (35g): GI= High, GL=High, Net carb= Varies

◼ Sweetened Dried Blueberries, ¼ cup (35g): GI= High, GL=High, Net carb= Varies

◼ Sweetened Dried Cherries, ¼ cup (40g): GI= High, GL=High, Net carb= Varies

◼ Sweetened Dried Cranberries, ¼ cup (40g): GI= High, GL=High, Net carb= Varies

◼ Sweetened Dried Mango, ¼ cup (40g): GI= High, GL=High, Net carb= Varies

▤ Sweetened Dried Peaches, ¼ cup (38g): GI= High, GL=High, Net carb= Varies

▤ Sweetened Dried Pears, ¼ cup (40g): GI= High, GL=High, Net carb= Varies

▤ Sweetened Dried Plums, ¼ cup (40g): GI= High, GL=High, Net carb= Varies

▤ Watermelon Jelly (store bought), 1 tbsp (20g): GI= High, GL=High, Net carb= Varies

MEATS - BEEF, LAMP, VEAL, PORK & POULTRY

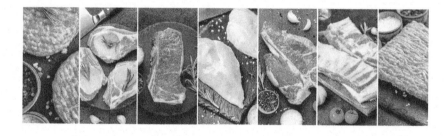

In the context of a T2D diet, it is important to be cautious about the types of meats consumed. While meat can be a valuable source of protein, vitamins, and minerals, certain considerations need to be made to align with the principles of a T2D diet.

- **High fat content:** Some cuts of meat, such as fatty cuts of beef, lamb, veal, pork, and poultry with visible skin, can contain high levels of unhealthy saturated fats. Consuming excessive amounts of these fats may contribute to insulin resistance.
- **Unhealthy cooking methods:** Meats that are prepared using unhealthy cooking methods, such as deep-frying or excessive breading, can lead to increased calorie and

unhealthy fat intake. These methods can elevate the risk of weight gain, high blood sugar levels, and other adverse health effects.

- **Processed meats:** Processed meats, including sausages, hot dogs, bacon, and deli meats, often contain additives, preservatives, and high levels of sodium. Frequent consumption of processed meats, including sausages, bacon, and ham, has been linked to an augmented likelihood of chronic conditions like diabetes, heart disease, and certain types of cancer, primarily colorectal cancer.
- **Portions and overall dietary balance:** Consuming excessive portions of meat can result in imbalanced meals and reduce the intake of other vital food groups, such as vegetables, whole grains, and legumes. These foods provide essential fiber, vitamins, and minerals necessary for maintaining overall health and blood sugar control.

It is essential to prioritize lean cuts of meat, trim visible fat, and choose healthier cooking methods like grilling, baking, or broiling. Additionally, incorporating plant-based protein sources and adopting a healthy diabetes diet that includes a variety of nutrient-rich foods can support better blood sugar control and overall health for individuals with T2D.

In the subsequent sections of this chapter, you will find specific categories of meats that do not align with the principles of a T2D diet.

SAUSAGES AND SIMILAR PROCESSED MEATS

Sausages and similar processed meats encompass a diverse range of products such as andouille sausage, bacon, bratwurst, chorizo, hot dogs, salami, and many more.

Non-Compliance with the DiabeteBalance Diet: These types of foods often do not conform to the principles of the DiabeteBalance Diet or the 2020-2025 Dietary Guidelines for Americans (DGA).

Processed meats like sausages usually have high sodium content and can be rich in saturated fats, both of which can contribute to elevated blood pressure and raise the probability of cardiovascular disease - two crucial health aspects that people with diabetes need to carefully manage.

In addition, processed meats may contain additives like nitrates and nitrites, which have been associated with various health issues. Furthermore, the protein content in these foods can be problematic for individuals with diabetes and Chronic Kidney Disease (CKD), as excessive protein intake can strain the kidneys. It is important for individuals with diabetes to be mindful of their food choices and limit their consumption of processed meats to support their overall health and well-being.

In terms of carbohydrates, some sausages and similar processed meats may contain fillers or flavorings that increase their sugar content, potentially leading to unpredictable effects on blood glucose levels.

Furthermore, these foods typically lack dietary fiber, an essential nutrient for regulating blood sugar levels and promoting overall digestive health.

Given their high sodium content, potential sugar content, lack of fiber, and potential health risks associated with certain additives, sausages and similar processed meats are generally not recommended for those seeking to better manage T2D. When making food choices, always scrutinize nutrition labels and aim to select fresh, minimally processed foods wherever possible.

The following is a list of items that are not suitable for individuals with diabetes:

▤ Andouille sausage ▤ Bacon ▤ BBQ sausage rolls ▤ Beef sausage rolls ▤ Black forest ham ▤ Black forest ham slices ▤ Black pudding ▤

Blood sausage ▤ Bockwurst ▤ Bologna ▤ Bratwurst ▤ Breakfast sausage links ▤ Breakfast sausage rolls ▤ Cajun-style sausage ▤ Cajun-style sausage (full-fat) ▤ Capicola ▤ Capicola slices ▤ Cervelat ▤ Cheese and sausage rolls ▤ Chicken sausage rolls ▤ Chicken sausages (commercially made) ▤ Chorizo ▤ Chorizo sausage rolls ▤ Classic pork sausage rolls ▤ Corned beef ▤ Corned venison ▤ Cured duck breast ▤ Deviled ham ▤ Duck confit ▤ Finnish sausage ▤ Frankfurters ▤ Genoa salami ▤ Goetta ▤ Ham (commercially made) ▤ Head cheese ▤ Honey-baked turkey (commercially made) ▤ Honey-glazed ham (commercially made) ▤ Honey-roasted ham (commercially made) ▤ Honey-smoked turkey (commercially made) ▤ Hot dogs ▤ Italian salami (full-fat) ▤ Italian sausage ▤ Italian sausage (regular) ▤ Kabanosy ▤ Kielbasa ▤ Lebanon bologna ▤ Linguica ▤ Liverwurst ▤ Lunch meats (e.g., turkey, chicken, roast beef) ▤ Merguez sausage ▤ Mortadella ▤ Mortadella slices ▤ Pastrami slices ▤ Peppered salami ▤ Pepperoni ▤ Pickled pork ▤ Polish sausage ▤ Potted meat ▤ Prosciutto slices ▤ Salami ▤ Sausages ▤ Smoked beef brisket ▤ Smoked beef ribs ▤ Smoked ham hock slices ▤ Smoked ham shank slices ▤ Smoked ham shoulder slices ▤ Smoked ham slices ▤ Smoked ham steak slices ▤ Smoked pork ribs ▤ Smoked sausages (full-fat) ▤ Smoked turkey/chicken breast ▤ Soppressata ▤ South African boerewors ▤ Summer sausage ▤ Thuringer sausage ▤ Turkey bacon ▤ Turkey pastrami ▤ Turkey roll ▤ Turkey sausage rolls ▤ Turkey sausages (commercially made) ▤ Vienna sausages ▤ Vienna sausages (full-fat) ▤ Weisswurst ▤ White pudding

BREADED AND DEEP-FRIED/BREADED AND FRIED FOODS

Breaded and deep-fried or simply fried foods include a wide variety of items such as breaded and fried cutlets of various meats, breaded and deep-fried chicken bites, and similar items.

Non-Compliance with the DiabeteBalance Diet: These foods typically do not align well with the principles of the DiabeteBalance Diet or the 2020-2025 Dietary Guidelines for Americans (DGA). They are often highly processed, high in unhealthy fats, and contain significant amounts of simple carbohydrates.

Breaded and fried foods are often high in trans and saturated fats due to the frying process. These fats can heighten the risk of heart disease, which individuals with diabetes are already at a higher risk of. Furthermore, the breading on these foods often contains refined flours with a high glycemic index (GI).

Moreover, these foods can be high in sodium, which can negatively impact blood pressure and cardiovascular health. The protein content in some of these foods can also pose a problem for individuals with diabetes and Chronic Kidney Disease (CKD) as excessive protein can strain the kidneys.

Additionally, breaded and fried foods often lack dietary fiber, which is essential for maintaining stable blood sugar levels and promoting overall digestive health.

Given their high GI, unhealthy fat content, and potential lack of key nutrients, breaded and deep-fried or fried foods are typically not the best choice for individuals trying to reverse T2D. As with any food choices, reading nutrition labels and prioritizing whole, unprocessed foods can make a significant difference in managing and improving health outcomes.

The following is a list of items that are not suitable for individuals with diabetes:

▤ Breaded and deep-fried chicken bites ▤ Breaded and deep-fried chicken breasts ▤ Breaded and deep-fried chicken chunks ▤ Breaded and deep-fried chicken cutlets ▤ Breaded and deep-fried chicken dippers ▤ Breaded and deep-fried chicken drumsticks ▤ Breaded and deep-fried chicken escalopes ▤ Breaded and deep-fried chicken fillets ▤ Breaded and deep-fried chicken fingers ▤ Breaded and deep-fried chicken fritters ▦ Breaded and deep-fried chicken goujons ▦ Breaded and deep-fried chicken lollipops ▦ Breaded and deep-fried chicken nuggets ▦ Breaded and deep-fried chicken patties ▦ Breaded and deep-fried chicken popcorn ▦ Breaded and deep-fried chicken strips ▦ Breaded and deep-fried chicken tenders ▦ Breaded and deep-fried chicken thighs ▦ Breaded and deep-fried chicken wings ▦ Breaded and fried beef cutlets ▦ Breaded and fried cauliflower cutlets ▦ Breaded and fried chicken cutlets ▦ Breaded and fried chicken schnitzel ▦ Breaded and fried clam cutlets ▦ Breaded and fried crab cutlets ▦ Breaded and fried eggplant cutlets ▦ Breaded and fried fish cutlets ▦ Breaded and fried lamb cutlets ▦ Breaded and fried lobster cutlets ▦ Breaded and fried mushroom cutlets ▦ Breaded and fried oyster cutlets ▦ Breaded and fried pork cutlets ▦ Breaded and fried pork schnitzel ▦ Breaded and fried potato cutlets ▦ Breaded and fried scallop cutlets ▦ Breaded and fried seitan cutlets ▦ Breaded and fried shrimp cutlets ▦ Breaded and fried tempeh cutlets ▦ Breaded and fried tofu cutlets ▦ Breaded and fried turkey cutlets ▦ Breaded and fried turkey schnitzel ▦ Breaded and fried veal cutlets ▦ Breaded and fried veal schnitzel ▦ Breaded and fried zucchini cutlets ▦ Breaded calamari rings ▦ Breaded clams ▦ Breaded clams ▦ Breaded crab cakes ▦ Breaded crab sticks ▦ Breaded fish cakes ▦ Breaded fish fillets ▦ Breaded fish fingers ▦ Breaded fish nuggets ▦ Breaded fish sandwiches ▦ Breaded fish sandwiches ▦ Breaded fish sticks ▦ Breaded lobster bites ▦ Breaded lobster bites ▦ Breaded oysters ▦ Breaded oysters ▦ Breaded scallops ▦ Breaded scallops ▦ Breaded shrimp ▦ Tempura-battered calamari ▦ Tempura-battered clams ▦ Tempura-battered crab sticks ▦ Tempura-battered fish ▦ Tempura-battered oysters ▦ Tempura-battered scallops ▦ Tempura-battered shrimp

Sliced Meats

Sliced meats, often used for sandwiches, include a variety of cold cuts, such as roast beef slices, ham slices, turkey slices, and other similar products.

Non-Compliance with the DiabeteBalance Diet: According to the principles of the DiabeteBalance Diet and the 2020-2025 Dietary Guidelines for Americans (DGA), sliced meats for sandwiches are generally discouraged. These products are typically processed, can contain high levels of sodium, and may include additives and preservatives.

Sliced meats' high sodium content can have detrimental effects on blood pressure and cardiovascular health, which is especially crucial for individuals with diabetes. In addition, the protein content in sliced meats could pose challenges for individuals managing T2D and Chronic Kidney Disease (CKD), as excessive protein consumption can overtax the kidneys.

Problematic Pairing with Bread: Sliced meats are often paired with bread to make sandwiches. However, many types of bread have a high Glycemic Index (GI), meaning they can rapidly raise blood sugar levels. This combination can be particularly problematic for individuals with T2D, as it can lead to increased carbohydrate intake and difficulty controlling blood sugar levels.

Furthermore, sliced meats and bread both typically lack significant amounts of dietary fiber. Fiber is essential for blood sugar regulation and digestive health, emphasizing these foods' unsuitability in a diet aimed at optimally managing diabetes.

While sliced meats can provide convenience, individuals aiming for T2D reversal should carefully consider their health impacts. Reading nutritional labels, making mindful dietary choices, and opting for whole, unprocessed foods whenever possible are vital steps in maintaining a balanced, health-promoting diet.

The following is a list of items that are not suitable for individuals with diabetes:

▤ Roast beef slices ▤ Turkey breast slices ▤ Ham slices ▤ Chicken breast slices ▤ Pastrami slices ▤ Corned beef slices ▤ Salami slices ▤ Pepperoni slices ▤ Prosciutto slices ▤ Mortadella slices ▤ Genoa salami slices ▤ Capicola slices ▤ Bologna slices ▤ Smoked turkey breast slices ▤ Smoked ham slices ▤ Smoked chicken breast slices ▤ Smoked salmon slices ▤ Smoked roast beef slices ▤ Smoked turkey/chicken breast slices ▤ Black forest ham slices ▤ Honey-roasted ham slices ▤ Honey-baked turkey slices ▤ Turkey pastrami slices ▤ Smoked bacon slices ▤ Roast lamb slices ▤ Roast pork slices ▤ Roast chicken slices ▤ Turkey pastrami slices ▤ Smoked chicken slices ▤ Smoked turkey slices ▤ Black forest ham slices ▤ Honey-roasted ham slices ▤ Roast lamb slices ▤ Roast pork slices ▤ Roast chicken slices ▤ Smoked bacon slices ▤ Turkey bacon slices ▤ Pancetta slices ▤ Canadian bacon slices ▤ Roast beef slices (seasoned/flavored variations) ▤ Turkey breast slices (seasoned/flavored variations) ▤ Ham slices (seasoned/flavored variations) ▤ Chicken breast slices (seasoned/flavored variations) ▤ Pastrami slices (seasoned/flavored variations) ▤ Corned beef slices (seasoned/flavored variations) ▤ Salami slices (seasoned/flavored variations) ▤ Pepperoni slices (seasoned/flavored variations) ▤ Prosciutto slices (seasoned/flavored variations) ▤ Mortadella slices (seasoned/flavored variations) ▤ Genoa salami slices (seasoned/flavored variations) ▤ Capicola slices (seasoned/flavored variations) ▤ Bologna slices (seasoned/flavored variations)

Canned/Preserved Meats:

Canned or preserved meats are products that have undergone preservation methods such as canning, curing, or drying to extend their shelf life and make them more convenient for storage and use. Examples include canned corned beef, canned roast beef, canned ham, canned pork, and other similar products.

Non-Compliance with the DiabeteBalance Diet: As per the principles of the DiabeteBalance Diet and the 2020-2025 Dietary Guidelines for Americans (DGA), the consumption of canned or preserved meats is generally not recommended. These products tend to be heavily processed, contain high levels of sodium, and often incorporate additives and preservatives.

Canned or preserved meats' high sodium content can negatively affect blood pressure and overall cardiovascular health, significant considerations for individuals with diabetes. Moreover, their protein content, while potentially beneficial in moderation, can be problematic for those managing T2D alongside Chronic Kidney Disease (CKD), as overconsumption of protein can put stress on the kidneys.

Additionally, some preserved meats may contain added sugars, which can contribute to higher carbohydrate intake and impact blood sugar levels. Pairing these meats with high Glycemic Index (GI) foods can lead to rapid increases in blood sugar levels, adding to the difficulty of effective T2D management.

Lastly, these products are typically low in dietary fiber, a crucial nutrient for blood sugar regulation and overall digestive health. This further limits their suitability in a diet aimed at reversing T2D.

Therefore, while canned and preserved meats may offer convenience, individuals aiming for T2D reversal should carefully consider their potential health impacts. Reading nutritional labels attentively and making mindful dietary choices are vital steps toward maintaining a balanced, healthful diet.

The following is a list of items that are not suitable for individuals with diabetes:

▣ Canned anchovies in oil ▣ Canned bacon ▣ Canned barbecue pork ▣ Canned beef chili ▣ Canned beef chunks ▣ Canned beef gravy ▣ Canned beef gravy mix ▣ Canned beef in BBQ sauce ▣ Canned beef in gravy ▣ Canned beef pot roast ▣ Canned beef pot roast with vegetables ▣ Canned beef ravioli ▣ Canned beef ravioli in tomato sauce ▣ Canned beef stew ▣ Canned beef stew with potatoes and carrots ▣ Canned beef stew with vegetables ▣ Canned beef stroganoff ▣ Canned beef tamales ▣ Canned chicken ▣ Canned chicken alfredo ▣ Canned chicken and dumplings ▣ Canned chicken and rice soup ▣ Canned chicken chunks ▣ Canned chicken curry ▣ Canned chicken gravy ▣ Canned chicken gravy mix ▣ Canned chicken in barbecue sauce ▣ Canned chicken in cream sauce ▣ Canned chicken noodle soup ▣ Canned chicken noodle soup with vegetables ▣ Canned chicken pot pie ▣ Canned chicken pot pie with vegetables ▣ Canned chicken salad ▣ Canned chicken spread ▣ Canned chicken tamales ▣ Canned chicken tikka masala ▣ Canned chili con carne ▣ Canned corned beef ▣ Canned corned beef hash ▣ Canned corned beef spread ▣ Canned corned mutton ▣ Canned deviled ham ▣ Canned duck confit ▣ Canned ham ▣ Canned ham slices ▣ Canned ham spread ▣ Canned hot dogs ▣ Canned liver pâté ▣ Canned luncheon meat ▣ Canned meat chili ▣ Canned meat curry ▣ Canned meat pies ▣ Canned meat sauce ▣ Canned meat tamales ▣ Canned meat tortellini ▣ Canned meat-based pasta sauce ▣ Canned meatballs ▣ Canned meatballs in sauce ▣ Canned meatloaf ▣ Canned mixed meat stew ▣ Canned pork ▣ Canned pork and beans ▣ Canned pork in gravy ▣ Canned pork shoulder ▣ Canned pork spread ▣ Canned potted meat ▣ Canned pulled pork ▣ Canned roast beef ▣ Canned roast beef slices ▣ Canned salmon in oil ▣ Canned sardines in oil ▣ Canned sausages in tomato sauce ▣ Canned spam ▣ Canned turkey ▣ Canned turkey breast slices ▣ Canned turkey chili ▣ Canned turkey chili with beans ▣ Canned turkey gravy ▣ Canned turkey gravy mix ▣ Canned turkey meatballs ▣ Canned turkey pot pie ▣ Canned turkey pot pie with vegetables ▣ Canned turkey spread ▣ Canned vienna sausages

Smoked Meats

Smoked meats include a variety of animal-based products, ranging from pork and beef to seafood such as catfish and clams. The smoking process, which involves curing the meat with smoke from burning or smoldering materials like wood, gives these products a distinctive flavor.

Non-Compliance with the DiabeteBalance Diet: The principles of the DiabeteBalance Diet, guided by the 2020-2025 Dietary Guidelines for Americans (DGA), typically discourage the consumption of smoked meats. These meats are processed and often high in sodium and additives, which could pose challenges for blood sugar management and overall health.

Though smoked meats may be an appealing choice for their distinct taste, their high sodium content can negatively impact blood pressure and cardiovascular health, both significant considerations for individuals with diabetes. Moreover, smoked meats, like any protein-rich food, consumed in large quantities can pose challenges for individuals managing diabetes alongside Chronic Kidney Disease (CKD). Over-consumption of protein can put stress on the kidneys and exacerbate CKD.

In addition, pairing smoked meats with high Glycemic Index (GI) foods can lead to sharp rises in blood glucose levels, presenting an additional concern for people with diabetes. High GI foods cause an abrupt spike in blood sugar levels, which can make it challenging to manage diabetes effectively.

It's essential for individuals aiming to better manage T2D to carefully consider the potential impacts of their food choices on their health. This involves being mindful of nutritional labels and being cautious about pairing high sodium or protein foods with high GI foods. Despite the flavor appeal of smoked meats, their nutritional profile may make them less suitable for a diet aimed at T2D reversal.

The following is a list of items that are not suitable for individuals with diabetes:

▤ Smoked andouille sausage ▤ Smoked bacon ▤ Smoked beef brisket ▤ Smoked beef jerky (non-fish varieties) ▤ Smoked beef ribs ▤

Smoked beef sausage ▤ Smoked beef tenderloin ▤ Smoked beef tri-tip ▤ Smoked bison ribs ▤ Smoked bison sausage ▤ Smoked bologna ▤ Smoked bratwurst ▤ Smoked chicken ▤ Smoked chicken breast ▤ Smoked chicken drumsticks ▤ Smoked chicken sausage ▤ Smoked chicken thighs ▤ Smoked chicken wings ▤ Smoked chorizo ▤ Smoked corned beef ▤ Smoked duck breast ▤ Smoked duck legs ▤ Smoked elk sausage ▤ Smoked elk tenderloin ▤ Smoked goat chops ▤ Smoked goat sausage ▤ Smoked goat shoulder ▤ Smoked goose breast ▤ Smoked ham ▤ Smoked ham hock ▤ Smoked ham shank ▤ Smoked ham slices ▤ Smoked ham steak ▤ Smoked hot dogs ▤ Smoked kangaroo steak ▤ Smoked lamb chops ▤ Smoked lamb leg ▤ Smoked lamb shoulder ▤ Smoked ostrich fillets ▤ Smoked pastrami ▤ Smoked pepperoni ▤ Smoked pheasant ▤ Smoked pork ▤ Smoked pork belly ▤ Smoked pork chops ▤ Smoked pork sausage ▤ Smoked pork shoulder ▤ Smoked pork tenderloin ▤ Smoked pulled pork ▤ Smoked quail ▤ Smoked rabbit ▤ Smoked salami ▤ Smoked sausage (e.g., smoked kielbasa, smoked bratwurst) ▤ Smoked sausage links (e.g., smoked breakfast sausage links) ▤ Smoked sausage patties (e.g., smoked breakfast sausage patties) ▤ Smoked turkey ▤ Smoked turkey bacon ▤ Smoked turkey breast ▤ Smoked turkey legs ▤ Smoked turkey sausage ▤ Smoked turkey wings ▤ Smoked venison jerky ▤ Smoked venison sausage ▤ Smoked venison tenderloin ▤ Smoked wild boar ribs ▤ Smoked wild boar sausage ▤ Smoked wild boar shoulder

Commercially Made/Processed Poultry

Commercially made or processed poultry items refer to chicken, turkey, and other poultry products that are mass-produced. These products, such as chicken nuggets, chicken patties, chicken tenders, and honey-baked turkey, often contain additives and preservatives and tend to be high in sodium.

Non-Compliance with the DiabeteBalance Diet: Consistent with

2020-2025 Dietary Guidelines for Americans (DGA) and principles of the DiabeteBalance Diet, commercially processed poultry products are generally not advised. These items are often prepared with unhealthy cooking methods, like deep-frying, and contain unhealthy additives that may hinder blood sugar management and overall health.

While commercially processed poultry products are quick and convenient, they pose potential health risks. Their high sodium content can negatively affect blood pressure and cardiovascular health, which is already a concern for those with diabetes. Moreover, these products often have added sugars, unhealthy fats, and other specific additives that can contribute to blood sugar fluctuations.

Additionally, for those managing diabetes along with Chronic Kidney Disease (CKD), consuming these high-protein foods in large amounts can strain the kidneys, potentially worsening CKD.

Therefore, despite their convenience, commercially processed poultry products may not be an optimal choice for individuals aiming to better manage T2D, especially those with additional health considerations like CKD. It's always prudent to review nutritional labels carefully and to consider the potential health impacts before integrating such foods into one's diet.

The following is a list of items that are not suitable for individuals with diabetes:

▤ Breaded chicken bites ▤ Breaded chicken burgers ▤ Breaded chicken cutlets ▤ Breaded chicken dippers ▤ Breaded chicken drumsticks ▤ Breaded chicken fillets ▤ Breaded chicken fingers ▤ Breaded chicken meatballs ▤ Breaded chicken popcorn ▤ Breaded chicken schnitzel ▤ Breaded chicken strips ▤ Breaded chicken wings ▤ Chicken nuggets ▤ Chicken patties ▤ Chicken tenders ▤ Grilled chicken breast strips ▤ Grilled chicken patties ▤ Grilled chicken tenders ▤ Grilled turkey breast slices ▤ Grilled turkey deli meat ▤ Honey-baked turkey ▤ Honey-glazed turkey ▤ Honey-roasted turkey

▤ Honey-smoked turkey ▤ Processed chicken burger patties ▤ Processed chicken deli meats (e.g., chicken ham) ▤ Processed chicken lunch meats (e.g., chicken bologna) ▤ Processed chicken meatballs ▤ Processed chicken sausages (e.g., chicken hot dogs) ▤ Processed turkey deli meats (e.g., turkey ham) ▤ Processed turkey lunch meats (e.g., turkey bologna) ▤ Processed turkey meatballs ▤ Processed turkey sausages (e.g., turkey hot dogs) ▤ Roasted chicken breast ▤ Roasted chicken slices ▤ Roasted turkey breast ▤ Roasted turkey slices ▤ Smoked turkey breast ▤ Smoked turkey deli meat ▤ Smoked turkey slices

Pies and Similar

Pies and similar products are prepared by filling a pastry crust with a variety of ingredients, then baking the mixture until it's ready to serve. This category includes an array of dishes like chicken and mushroom pies, chicken pot pies, cottage pie, curry meat pies, lamb meat pies, shepherd's pie, steak and kidney pies, tourtière, turkey pot pies, and vegetable and meat pies.

Non-Compliance with the DiabeteBalance Diet: According to 2020-2025 Dietary Guidelines for Americans (DGA) and the principles of the DiabeteBalance Diet, foods like pies are typically not recommended. They are often made with refined flour and contain additives that may interfere with blood sugar management and overall health. Furthermore, the filling may have high levels of fat and salt, and sometimes even added sugars.

While pies may seem like a comforting meal option, their high carbohydrate content from the pastry crust, potential for added sugars, and high fat content can pose challenges for individuals with diabetes. This is especially the case for those also dealing with CKD, as the high protein content in meat-based pies can put additional strain on already compromised kidneys.

DR. H. MAHER

Thus, despite their convenience and taste appeal, pies may not be the best choice for individuals trying to better manage T2D, particularly those with additional health concerns like CKD. As always, it's advisable to read nutritional labels carefully and to take potential health impacts into account before incorporating such foods into one's diet.

The following is a list of items that are not suitable for individuals with diabetes:

Beef and ale pies ▤ Beef and Guinness pies ▤ Beef and mushroom pies ▤ Beef and onion pies ▤ Beef and Stilton pies ▤ Beef and vegetable pies ▤ Chicken and asparagus pies ▤ Chicken and bacon pies ▤ Chicken and chorizo pies ▤ Chicken and ham pies ▤ Chicken and leek pies ▤ Chicken and mushroom pies ▤ Chicken and spinach pies ▤ Chicken and sweetcorn pies ▤ Chicken and vegetable pies ▤ Chicken pot pies ▤ Cottage pie ▤ Curry meat pies ▤ Lamb and mint pies ▤ Lamb and potato pies ▤ Lamb and rosemary pies ▤ Lamb and vegetable pies ▤ Lamb meat pies ▤ Mushroom and leek pies ▤ Mushroom and Stilton pies ▤ Mushroom and tarragon pies ▤ Pork and apple pies ▤ Pork and black pudding pies ▤ Pork and sage pies ▤ Shepherd's pie ▤ Spinach and feta pies ▤ Spinach and mushroom pies ▤ Steak and kidney pies ▤ Tourtière ▤ Turkey and cranberry pies ▤ Turkey and ham pies ▤ Turkey and stuffing pies ▤ Turkey pot pies ▤ Vegetable and meat pies ▤ Vegetarian pies (e.g., vegetable pie, cheese and onion pie)

Jerkies

Jerky is a type of lean meat that undergoes a process of fat trimming, slicing into strips, and then drying to prevent spoilage. The drying process typically involves the addition of salt to inhibit the growth of bacteria on the meat until enough moisture has been removed.

Non-Compliance with The DiabeteBalance Diet: As per the 2020-2025 Dietary Guidelines for Americans and the principles of the the

DiabeteBalance Diet, processed foods like jerky are generally not recommended. They often lack key nutrients and contain additives that can interfere with blood sugar management and overall health.

Thus, while jerky might seem like a convenient source of protein, its high sodium and protein content, along with potential added sugars and lack of fiber, make it less suitable for people with diabetes, particularly those also dealing with CKD. Always read the nutritional labels carefully and consider the potential impacts on your health before including it in your diet.

The following is a list of items that are not suitable for individuals with diabetes:

▤ Alligator jerky ▤ BBQ pork jerky ▤ Beef jerky ▤ Bison jerky ▤ Cajun-style alligator jerky ▤ Carolina Reaper hot pepper beef jerky ▤ Chicken jerky ▤ Chicken teriyaki jerky ▤ Chipotle pork jerky ▤ Citrus teriyaki salmon jerky ▤ Cranberry maple elk jerky ▤ Elk jerky ▤ Garlic and black pepper beef jerky ▤ Hickory-smoked venison jerky ▤ Honey mustard chicken jerky ▤ Honey sriracha buffalo jerky ▤ Honey-glazed turkey jerky ▤ Kangaroo jerky ▤ Lemon pepper turkey jerky ▤ Maple brown sugar bacon jerky ▤ Maple-glazed bacon jerky ▤ Ostrich jerky ▤ Peppered beef jerky ▤ Peppered venison jerky ▤ Pork jerky ▤ Salmon jerky ▤ Sesame ginger turkey jerky ▤ Smoked salmon jerky ▤ Smoky barbecue bison jerky ▤ Smoky mesquite trout jerky ▤ Spicy buffalo jerky ▤ Sriracha chicken jerky ▤ Sweet and spicy jerky ▤ Sweet mesquite pork jerky ▤ Teriyaki kangaroo jerky ▤ Teriyaki venison jerky ▤ Trout jerky ▤ Tuna jerky ▤ Turkey jerky ▤ Venison jerky

High Fat Ground Meats

High fat ground meats include products such as fatty ground turkey, ground lamb with a higher fat percentage, ground pork with a higher fat percentage, and ground veal with a higher fat percentage.

Non-Compliance with the DiabeteBalance Diet: Ground meats with high fat content are typically not recommended as per the 2020-2025 Dietary Guidelines for Americans and the principles of the Diabete-Balance Diet.

Highly fatty meats, particularly when they are processed or cooked in unhealthy ways, can lead to excessive intake of saturated fats. This can contribute to higher cholesterol levels, increased risk of heart disease, and weight gain, all of which are health concerns for individuals managing diabetes.

Moreover, the protein content of these ground meats can also be problematic for those with diabetes and Chronic Kidney Disease (CKD), as excessive protein consumption can exacerbate kidney function issues.

The fact that these are ground meats also often means they've been mechanically processed, which can sometimes involve the use of additives and preservatives that aren't conducive to the DiabeteBalance Diet.

These meats generally lack fiber and can be paired with high Glycemic Index (GL) foods, such as bread or pasta, leading to potential spikes in blood sugar levels.

Thus, high fat ground meats can pose various challenges in the management and potential reversal of T2D. Whenever possible, choose lean cuts of fresh meat over high-fat or processed options, and consider pairing them with low GL foods for optimal blood glucose control.

The following is a list of items that are not suitable for individuals with diabetes:

▤ Ground beef (regular or high-fat) ▤ Ground pork ▤ Ground lamb ▤ Ground veal ▤ Ground duck ▤ Ground goose ▤ Ground bison ▤ Ground sausage (various flavors) ▤ Ground chorizo ▤ Ground fatty cuts of beef, such as chuck or brisket (when ground) ▤ Ground fatty cuts of pork, such as shoulder or belly (when ground) ▤ Ground fatty cuts of lamb, such as shoulder or leg (when ground) ▤ Ground fatty cuts of veal, such as shoulder or rib (when ground) ▤ Ground fatty cuts of duck, such as leg or breast (when ground) ▤ Ground fatty cuts of goose, such as leg or breast (when ground) ▤ Ground fatty cuts of bison, such as chuck or rib (when ground) ▤ Ground fatty cuts of turkey, such as thigh or dark meat (when ground) ▤ Ground fatty cuts of chicken, such as thigh or dark meat (when ground) ▤ Ground fatty cuts of game meats (when ground) ▤ Ground fatty cuts of other animal meats, such as rabbit or kangaroo (when ground)

Other Processed Meats

"Other Processed Meats" is a category that encompasses a variety of meat products, including Black pudding, Blood sausage, Corned beef, Corned venison, Duck confit, Head cheese, Liverwurst, etc.

Non-Compliance with the DiabeteBalance Diet: The 2020-2025 Dietary Guidelines for Americans (DGA) and the principles of the DiabeteBalance Diet discourage the consumption of highly processed meats.

These kinds of processed meats often contain additives, preservatives, and are typically high in sodium, all of which can negatively impact blood sugar management and overall health in people with diabetes.

Similar to other processed meats, these products can also be high in fat and protein. Excessive intake of fats, particularly saturated and trans fats, can contribute to elevated cholesterol levels, and increased risk of heart disease. On the other hand, excessive protein can be a concern for individuals with diabetes and Chronic Kidney Disease (CKD), as it can exacerbate kidney function issues.

These meats also tend to lack fiber, a key nutrient that can help regulate blood sugar levels and support overall digestive health.

Additionally, these types of processed meats are often consumed in combination with high Glycemic Index (GL) foods, which can lead to sudden spikes in blood sugar levels.

Therefore, while these "other processed meats" might be appealing for their unique flavors and convenience, their potential negative health impacts make them less suitable for those seeking to better manage T2D. Instead, focus on fresh, minimally processed meats and pair them with low GL foods for better blood glucose control.

The following is a list of items that are not suitable for individuals with diabetes:

▤ Black pudding ▤ Blood sausage ▤ Corned beef ▤ Corned venison ▤ Duck confit ▤ Head cheese ▤ Liverwurst ▤ Mortadella ▤ Pancetta ▤ Pastrami ▤ Pepperoni ▤ Prosciutto ▤ Salami (various types such as Genoa, Milano, or Soppressata) ▤ Sausage (various types such as Italian, bratwurst, or breakfast sausage) ▤ Smoked ham ▤ Smoked turkey ▤ Smoked salmon ▤ Spam (canned meat product) ▤ Summer sausage ▤ Vienna sausage

NUTS AND SEEDS

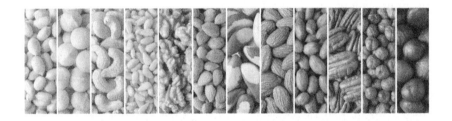

Here are some categories that do not comply with the diet's principles.

HONEY-ROASTED OR SUGARED NUTS

Nuts are generally a nutritious snack option, packed with beneficial fats, protein, and fiber. However, when they're honey-roasted or coated with sugar, they become far less suitable for individuals following the DiabeteBalance Diet.

Non-Compliance with the DiabeteBalance Diet: Honey-roasted or sugared nuts typically don't align with the principles of the Diabete-

Balance Diet and the 2020-2025 Dietary Guidelines for Americans (DGA).

When nuts are honey-roasted or coated with sugar, their carbohydrate and sugar content experiences a significant increase. These additional sugars can cause a rapid surge in blood sugar levels, which poses a challenge for individuals with diabetes or those aiming to reverse T2D.

Moreover, the roasting procedure may involve the use of unhealthy oils, resulting in an elevated intake of unhealthy fats. Consuming excessive amounts of unhealthy fats can contribute to weight gain and other health illnesses, including heart disease.

Furthermore, the added sugars and flavors can make these nuts more palatable and potentially lead to overeating, which can further promote weight gain – a factor that can worsen insulin resistance and hinder the process of reversing T2D.

Given their high sugar content and the potential for overeating, honey-roasted or sugared nuts are typically not the best choice for individuals managing or trying to reverse T2D. Opt instead for unsweetened, raw, or dry-roasted nuts, which provide the nutritional benefits of nuts without the added sugars. Always remember to pay attention to portion sizes, as even the healthiest of nuts are calorie-dense.

The following is a list of items that are not suitable for individuals with diabetes:

▤ Candied almonds ▤ Candied cashews ▤ Candied peanuts ▤ Candied pecans ▤ Candied pistachios ▤ Candied walnuts ▤ Frosted almonds ▤ Frosted cashews ▤ Frosted peanuts ▤ Frosted pecans ▤ Frosted pistachios ▤ Frosted walnuts ▤ Glazed almonds ▤ Glazed cashews ▤ Glazed peanuts ▤ Glazed pecans ▤ Glazed pistachios ▤ Glazed walnuts ▤ Honey-roasted almonds ▤ Honey-roasted cashews ▤ Honey-roasted peanuts ▤ Honey-roasted pecans ▤ Honey-roasted pistachios ▤ Honey-roasted walnuts ▤ Sugared almonds ▤ Sugared cashews ▤ Sugared peanuts ▤ Sugared pecans ▤ Sugared pistachios ▤ Sugared walnuts

---

SWEETENED NUT BUTTERS

While nut butters can be a good source of healthy fats and protein, those that have added sugars or sweeteners can contribute to elevated blood sugar levels, making them less suitable for individuals following the DiabeteBalance Diet.

Non-Compliance with the DiabeteBalance Diet: Sweetened nut butters often conflict with the principles of the DiabeteBalance Diet and the 2020-2025 Dietary Guidelines for Americans (DGA).

Nut butters (e.g., peanut butter, almond butter, cashew butter) can be part of a healthy diet due to their high protein and healthy fat content. However, when sweeteners or sugars are added, these otherwise healthy options can become problematic for individuals managing T2D. The added sugars increase the overall carbohydrate content, potentially causing spikes in blood sugar levels.

These products can also contribute to weight gain when consumed in excess, particularly because the added sweetness can make them easy to overeat. Weight management is crucial for those with T2D, as it can directly impact insulin sensitivity and overall blood glucose control.

Furthermore, sweetened nut butters often contain unhealthy oils and additives, detracting from their nutritional benefits.

Given the potential negative effects on blood sugar control and weight management, sweetened nut butters are not the best choice for those seeking to better manage T2D. It's recommended to opt for natural, unsweetened varieties of nut butters and pay close attention to portion sizes due to their raised calorie content.

The following is a list of items that are not suitable for individuals with diabetes:

▤ Blueberry muffin peanut butter ▤ Brownie batter peanut butter ▤ Butter toffee almond butter ▤ Caramel apple pecan butter ▤ Cherry almond butter ▤ Chocolate banana hazelnut spread ▤ Chocolate chip cookie dough peanut butter ▤ Chocolate coconut almond butter ▤ Chocolate hazelnut spread ▤ Chocolate mint cashew butter ▤ Chocolate raspberry hazelnut spread ▤ Cinnamon raisin peanut butter ▤ Cinnamon swirl peanut butter ▤ Coconut chocolate chip almond butter ▤ Coconut cookie dough peanut butter ▤ Coconut maple pecan butter ▤ Cookie butter spread ▤ Cookies and cream almond butter ▤ Espresso almond butter ▤ Gingerbread spice almond butter ▤ Graham cracker almond butter ▤ Honey roasted cashew butter ▤ Honey roasted walnut butter ▤ Honey vanilla cashew butter ▤ Honey-flavored peanut butter ▤ Maple pecan almond butter ▤ Maple walnut butter ▤ Maple-flavored almond butter ▤ Marshmallow-flavored peanut butter ▤ Mocha hazelnut spread ▤ Mocha java almond butter ▤ Mocha-flavored almond butter ▤ Peanut butter cookie dough almond butter ▤ Peppermint chocolate hazelnut spread ▤ Pumpkin pie spiced peanut butter ▤ Pumpkin spice almond butter ▤ Salted caramel almond butter ▤ Salted caramel macadamia nut butter ▤ Salted caramel peanut butter ▤ Salted caramel pecan butter ▤ Salted toffee peanut butter ▤ Snickerdoodle cashew butter ▤ Strawberry shortcake almond butter ▤ Sweetened cinnamon almond butter ▤ Vanilla caramel cashew butter ▤ Vanilla chai cashew butter ▤ Vanilla-flavored cashew butter ▤ White chocolate macadamia nut butter

SUGARED OR GLAZED SEEDS

While seeds are generally a good source of healthy fats, fiber, and essential nutrients, when they're coated with sugar or a glaze, their carbohydrate and added sugar content can rise significantly, making them less appropriate for individuals following the DiabeteBalance Diet.

Non-Compliance with the DiabeteBalance Diet: Sugared or glazed seeds often conflict with the principles of the DiabeteBalance Diet and the 2020-2025 Dietary Guidelines for Americans (DGA).

Seeds, such as pumpkin, sunflower, or flax seeds, naturally have a balanced profile of protein, healthy fats, and fiber, which aids in blood sugar regulation. However, the addition of a sugary coating increases their carbohydrate content, potentially leading to spikes in blood sugar levels.

Moreover, sugared or glazed seeds can contribute to weight gain if consumed excessively due to their elevated calorie content. Weight management is crucial in controlling and optimally managing diabetes because it directly influences insulin sensitivity and overall glucose management.

In addition to sugar, these products may contain unhealthy oils and additives, which further decrease their nutritional value.

Due to their potential impact on blood sugar control and weight management, sugared or glazed seeds aren't the most beneficial option for those aiming to better manage T2D. Instead, it's advised to select plain seeds and to be aware of portion sizes due to their high calorie content.

The following is a list of items that are not suitable for individuals with diabetes:

▤ Candied sunflower seeds ▤ Caramel-covered pepitas (pumpkin seeds) ▤ Caramelized pepitas (pumpkin seeds) ▤ Chocolate-covered flaxseeds ▤ Cinnamon-glazed sunflower kernels ▤ Cinnamon-sugar coated sesame seeds ▤ Coconut-coated chia seeds ▤ Frosted flaxseeds ▤ Frosted hemp seeds ▤ Glazed sesame seeds ▤ Honey-coated flaxseeds ▤ Honey-glazed pumpkin seeds ▤ Honey-roasted sunflower kernels ▤ Honeyed poppy seeds ▤ Maple-coated sesame seeds ▤ Maple-flavored poppy seeds ▤ Sugared pumpkin seeds ▤ Sugared sunflower kernels ▤ Sweetened chia seeds ▤ Sweetened hemp seeds

OIL, FAT AND CONDIMENTS

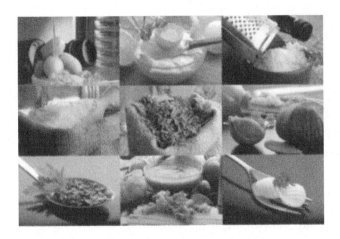

Effective management of diabetes necessitate a comprehensive and nuanced approach to dietary choices. This doesn't merely involve the total quantity of fats and oils consumed, but also encapsulates the quality of those fats, their sources, and the cooking techniques employed. Certain oils, fats, and condiments have properties that can exert a negative influence on blood sugar levels, weight control, and overall health. Understanding these intricacies is vital in the journey toward optimal T2D management.

NON-COMPLIANT OILS AND FATS:

Palm and Coconut oils, along with Lard, are high in saturated fats. Regular consumption of these can negatively affect cholesterol levels, insulin sensitivity, and increase the risk of heart disease. Vegetable shortening and some margarine products contain trans fats, which have been directly linked to heart disease.

Grapeseed and Cottonseed oils, rich in polyunsaturated fats, contain a high omega-6 fatty acid content. The disproportionate ratio of omega-6 to omega-3 fatty acids can result in inflammation, which poses a risk factor for chronic conditions like T2D. Processed foods such as pastries and snacks often contain hydrogenated or partially hydrogenated oils, which harbor detrimental trans fats.

Animal-based fats, especially those derived from red and processed meats, have elevated levels of saturated fats and cholesterol. Fat drippings from processed meats like sausages or bacon are also high in unhealthy fats.

Cooking methods matter too. Deep frying can contribute to the creation of Advanced Glycation End-products (AGEs), which have been linked to chronic ailments (e.g, diabetes and heart disease). Also, frying oils can surpass their smoke point, making the oil toxic and harmful to health.

Switching to oils high in monounsaturated and polyunsaturated fats, like olive oil, avocado oil, and canola oil, can be beneficial. These oils align with the principles of the DiabeteBalance Diet, contributing to improved heart health.

Remember, while fats are an essential part of our diet, it's the type of fat that matters. Prioritize unsaturated fats over saturated and trans fats, consider the smoke point when cooking, and monitor the (omega-6, omega-3) ratio in your diet.

NON-COMPLIANT CONDIMENTS:

Many condiments, despite being used in small quantities, can be high in sugars, unhealthy fats, or sodium, which may not align with the DiabeteBalance Diet.

Examples of such condiments include:

- Ketchup, barbecue sauce, and sweet chili sauce, which often contain high amounts of added sugars.
- Mayonnaise and some salad dressings, high in unhealthy fats.
- Soy sauce, pickles, and other pickled or brined condiments, which can contain high levels of sodium.
- Teriyaki sauce: Teriyaki sauce often contains a significant amount of added sugars, which can negatively impact blood sugar levels. Look for low-sugar or sugar-free alternatives.
- Sweet and sour sauce: Similar to teriyaki sauce, sweet and sour sauce is high in added sugars. Choose options with reduced or no sugar.
- Honey mustard: While mustard itself is generally a healthier choice, honey mustard often contains added sugars. Opt for regular mustard or make your own sugar-free version.
- Barbecue and marinade sauces: Many barbecue and marinade sauces are loaded with sugar and can contribute to elevated blood sugar levels. Look for low-sugar or sugar-free options, or consider making your own using natural sweeteners in moderation.
- Syrups and toppings: Maple syrup, chocolate syrup, and other dessert toppings are high in sugars. Avoid or limit their use in your the DiabeteBalance Diet.
- Relish: Some commercial relish products can contain added sugars and high amounts of sodium. Choose sugar-free or homemade relish options.

Remember to carefully read food labels when purchasing condiments, as ingredients and nutritional content can vary among brands. Opting for homemade versions or using herbs, spices, and vinegar-based dressings can help you avoid unnecessary sugars, unhealthy fats, and excessive sodium.

VEGETABLES AND VEGETABLE PRODUCTS

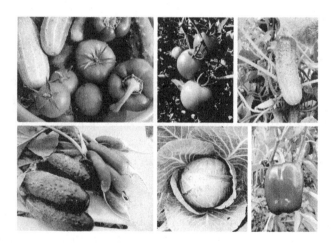

While vegetables are a cornerstone of a balanced diet and lauded for their health benefits, certain cooking techniques can morph these nutritional stalwarts into less healthy options, particularly for individuals managing T2D. Let's discuss several such methods that cause vegetables to fall outside the DiabeteBalance Diet's compliance.

- Deep-Frying: Deep-frying is a primary culprit that can turn a wholesome vegetable into a less healthy choice. Unhealthy fats often used in deep-frying can spur weight gain, inflammation, and insulin resistance, rendering vegetables like broccoli, zucchini, or cauliflower, less nutritionally beneficial.

- Addition of Sugars or Sweetening Agents: The introduction of sugars or sweetening agents such as honey during vegetable preparation can also create non-compliance. This includes applying high sugar-content glazes or marinades to vegetables like carrots, bell peppers, or Brussels sprouts. High sugar intake correlates with raised blood glucose levels and elevated risks of T2D complications.
- Utilizing Creamy or Sugary Sauces: Dousing vegetables in creamy or sugary sauces, like cheese sauces, cream-based dressings, or sweet chili sauces, is inadvisable. These sauces often harbor high levels of unhealthy fats and added sugars, potentially increasing the glycemic load (GL) and causing blood glucose spikes.
- Breading or Batter Coating: Enveloping vegetables in a shell of breading or batter, as seen in tempura vegetables or onion rings, can also transition them into non-compliant foods. These coverings, typically made from high GI processed flours and often deep-fried, further amplify unhealthy fat content.
- Excessive Use of Unhealthy Fats: Preparing vegetables with an overabundance of unhealthy fats, such as butter, cheese, or heavy cream, can also render them non-compliant. Instances include scalloped potatoes, green bean casserole, or broccoli in cheese sauce.

STARCHY VEGETABLES AND BAKING:

Baking, particularly with starchy vegetables, concerns those managing blood sugar levels due to the possible impact on the foods' glycemic index (GI). The heat of baking can break down the vegetable's cellular structure, making its carbohydrates more readily digestible, and potentially causing a higher glycemic response.

This process, known as gelatinization, can elevate the GI of starchy foods like potatoes when baked. However, most vegetables, particularly non-starchy ones such as broccoli, cauliflower, Brussels sprouts, and leafy greens, naturally have a low GI. The fiber in these foods can decelerate carbohydrate digestion and absorption, mitigating blood sugar spikes.

Cooking methods preserving more of the vegetable's natural moisture, such as steaming or light sautéing, might impact the GI less than high-temperature baking. It's also worth noting that the effect of a food's GI on blood sugar levels can be moderated by what it's paired with – incorporating protein, healthy fats, and additional fiber can stabilize blood sugar levels.

Even as vegetables play a critical role in a balanced diet, it's crucial to prepare them in a manner that retains their nutritional value and aligns with health goals. By steering clear of the above preparation techniques, you can ensure that your vegetables align with the DiabeteBalance Diet.

Here is an exhaustive list of non-compliant vegetables or vegetable products:

▦ Balsamic Glazed Grilled Red Onions ▦ Broccoli with Cheese Sauce ▦ Broccoli with Cheese Sauce ▦ Candied Sweet Potatoes ▦ Cauliflower in Cheese Sauce ▦ Cauliflower in Cheese Sauce ▦ Corn Casserole ▦ Corn Casserole ▦ Corn on the cob with butter and/or sugar ▦ Corn on the cob with butter and/or sugar ▦ Creamed Corn ▦ Creamed Corn ▦ Creamed Spinach ▦ Creamed Spinach ▦ Creamy Asparagus ▦ Creamy Asparagus ▦ Creamy Coleslaw ▦ Creamy Coleslaw ▦ Creamy Corn ▦ Creamy Corn ▦ Creamy Potato Salad ▦ Creamy Potato Salad ▦ French Fries ▦ Fried Artichoke Hearts ▦ Fried Artichoke Hearts ▦ Fried Asparagus ▦ Fried Asparagus ▦ Fried Avocado Slices ▦ Fried Avocado Slices ▦ Fried Broccoli ▦ Fried

Broccoli ▦ Fried Brussels Sprouts ▦ Fried Brussels Sprouts ▦ Fried Cauliflower ▦ Fried Cauliflower ▦ Fried Corn Nuggets ▦ Fried Corn Nuggets ▦ Fried Eggplant ▦ Fried Eggplant ▦ Fried Green Beans ▦ Fried Green Beans ▦ Fried Green Tomatoes ▦ Fried Green Tomatoes ▦ Fried Jalapeno Poppers ▦ Fried Jalapeno Poppers ▦ Fried Mushrooms ▦ Fried Mushrooms ▦ Fried Okra ▦ Fried Okra ▦ Fried Pickles ▦ Fried Pickles ▦ Fried Plantains ▦ Fried Plantains ▦ Fried Sweet Potato Fries ▦ Fried Sweet Potato Fries ▦ Fried Tofu ▦ Fried Tofu ▦ Fried Zucchini ▦ Fried Zucchini ▦ General Tso's Vegetables ▦ General Tso's Vegetables ▦ Glazed Carrots ▦ Glazed Carrots ▦ Green Bean Casserole ▦ Green Bean Casserole ▦ Grilled Lemon-Honey Glazed Zucchini ▦ Grilled Lemon-Honey Glazed Zucchini ▦ Grilled Pineapple with Brown Sugar Glaze ▦ Grilled Pineapple with Brown Sugar Glaze ▦ Grilled Soy-Ginger Glazed Eggplant ▦ Grilled Soy-Ginger Glazed Eggplant ▦ Grilled Sweet and Spicy Glazed Corn on the Cob ▦ Grilled Sweet and Spicy Glazed Corn on the Cob ▦ Grilled Sweet Chili Glazed Bell Peppers ▦ Grilled Sweet Chili Glazed Bell Peppers ▦ Grilled Teriyaki Glazed Vegetables ▦ Grilled Teriyaki Glazed Vegetables ▦ Grilled vegetables with a high-sugar glaze or marinade ▦ Honey-Glazed Brussels Sprouts ▦ Honey-Glazed Brussels Sprouts ▦ Honey-Glazed Grilled Carrots ▦ Honey-Glazed Grilled Carrots ▦ Kung Pao Vegetables ▦ Kung Pao Vegetables ▦ Maple-Glazed Grilled Sweet Potatoes ▦ Maple-Glazed Grilled Sweet Potatoes ▦ Mashed Potatoes with heavy cream and butter ▦ Onion Rings ▦ Orange-Glazed Grilled Brussels Sprouts ▦ Orange-Glazed Grilled Brussels Sprouts ▦ Peas and Carrots with added sugar ▦ Potato Gratin with cream and cheese ▦ Potato Pancakes ▦ Potatoes Au Gratin ▦ Scalloped Potatoes ▦ Sweet and Sour Cabbage ▦ Sweet and Sour Cabbage ▦ Sweet and Sour Vegetables ▦ Sweet and Sour Vegetables ▦ Sweet Chili Vegetable Stir-fry ▦ Sweet Chili Vegetable Stir-fry ▦ Sweet Glazed Carrots ▦ Sweet Glazed Carrots ▦ Sweet Maple Glazed Beets ▦ Sweet Maple Glazed Beets ▦ Sweet Potato Casserole with marshmallows and brown sugar ▦ Szechuan Vegetables ▦ Szechuan Vegetables ▦ Tempura Vegetables ▦ Tempura Vegetables ▦ Teriyaki Vegetables ▦ Teriyaki Vegetables ▦ Vegetable

Chow Mein ▤ Vegetable Chow Mein ▤ Vegetable Fried Rice ▤ Vegetable Fried Rice ▤ Vegetable Lo Mein ▤ Vegetable Lo Mein ▤ Vegetables in creamy or sugary sauces ▤ Vegetables in creamy or sugary sauces

---

In the following section of this chapter, you'll find a detailed list that outline foods deemed non-compliant with the DiabeteBalance Diet. This list provide in-depth information, including serving size, Glycemic Index (GI), Glycemic Load (GL), and Net Carbohydrates for each listed food. These factors are particularly significant when food items are considered non-compliant due to their high glycemic load and/or substantial carbohydrate content.

However, it's important to remember that not all non-compliant foods fall into this category strictly based on their GI, GL, or net carbohydrate metrics. Certain food items are designated non-compliant due to other factors, such as intensive processing, excessive sodium content, or a high concentration of unhealthy fats. In these instances, the list may not provide detailed GI, GL, or net carbohy-drate data for these specific foods. Instead, these items will be listed with a clear annotation marking them as non-compliant. This distinc-tion is intended to enhance clarity about why certain foods are not advised within the framework of the DiabeteBalance Diet.

▤ Baked Beans, canned, ½ cup (130 g): GI= High, GL= High, Net carb= 27g

▤ Baked Russet Potatoes, 1 medium (173 g): GI= High, GL= High, Net carb= 37g

▤ Balsamic Glazed Grilled Red Onions, ½ cup (115 g): GI= High, GL=High, Net carb= Varies

▤ Beet Juice, 1 cup (250 ml): GI= High, GL= High, Net carb= 25g

▤ Beets, canned, ½ cup (85 g): GI= High, GL= High, Net carb= 16g

▤ Boiled Broad Beans, ½ cup (88 g): GI= High, GL= High, Net carb= 16g

▤ Boiled Yam, 1 cup (136 g): GI= High, GL= High, Net carb= 37g

▤ Breaded Cauliflower, fried, 1 cup (180 g): GI= High, GL= High, Net carb= 23g

▤ Candied Sweet Potatoes, ½ cup (115 g): GI= High, GL=High, Net carb= Varies

▤ Canned Mixed Vegetables, 1 cup (175 g): GI= High, GL= High, Net carb= 17g

▤ Carrot Cake, 1 slice (78 g): GI= High, GL= High, Net carb= 33g

▤ Carrot Juice, 1 cup (250 ml): GI= High, GL= High, Net carb= 22g

▤ Corn Chips, 1 oz (28 g): GI= High, GL= High, Net carb= 15g

▤ Corn Chowder, 1 cup (248 g): GI= High, GL= High, Net carb= 21g

▤ Corn Muffin, 1 medium (57 g): GI= High, GL= High, Net carb= 28g

▤ Corn Pasta, cooked, 1 cup (140 g): GI= High, GL= High, Net carb= 43g

▤ Corn Polenta, 1 cup (160 g): GI= High, GL= High, Net carb= 24g

▤ Corn Pudding, 1 cup (250 g): GI= High, GL= High, Net carb= 30g

▤ Corn Tamale, 1 tamale (186 g): GI= High, GL= High, Net carb= 45g

▤ Corn Tortillas, 2 tortillas (50 g): GI= High, GL= High, Net carb= 22g

▤ Cornbread Dressing, 1 cup (200 g): GI= High, GL= High, Net carb= 32g

▤ Cornbread Stuffing, 1 cup (200 g): GI= High, GL= High, Net carb= 38g

▤ Cornbread, 1 piece (60 g): GI= High, GL= High, Net carb= 21g

▤ Corned Beef Hash, canned, 1 cup (236 g): GI= High, GL= High, Net carb= 27g

▤ Creamed Corn, canned, ½ cup (125 g): GI= High, GL= High, Net carb= 21g

▤ French Fries, ½ cup (115 g): GI= High, GL=High, Net carb= Varies

▤ French Fries, fast food, ½ cup (74 g): GI= High, GL= High, Net carb= 23g

▤ Fried Eggplant, breaded, 1 cup (99 g): GI= High, GL= High, Net carb= 16g

▤ Fried Okra, ½ cup (100 g): GI= High, GL= High, Net carb= 15g

▤ Fried Zucchini, breaded, 1 cup (124 g): GI= High, GL= High, Net carb= 20g

▤ Grilled Corn on the Cob with Butter, 1 medium (200 g): GI= High, GL= High, Net carb= 24g

▤ Hash Browns, 1 cup (156 g): GI= High, GL= High, Net carb= 31g

▤ Instant Mashed Potatoes, 1 cup (210 g): GI= High, GL= High, Net carb= 36g

▤ Mashed Potatoes, 1 cup (210 g): GI= High, GL= High, Net carb= 36g

▤ Onion Rings, breaded and fried, 10 rings (83 g): GI= High, GL= High, Net carb= 31g

▤ Parsnips, boiled, ½ cup (78 g): GI= High, GL= High, Net carb= 14g

▤ Potato Chips, 1 oz (28 g): GI= High, GL= High, Net carb= 15g

▤ Potato Croquettes, 2 pieces (70 g): GI= High, GL= High, Net carb= 15g

▤ Potato Gnocchi, 1 cup (160 g): GI= High, GL= High, Net carb= 33g

▤ Potato Pancakes, 1 pancake (65 g): GI= High, GL= High, Net carb= 13g

▤ Potato Salad, 1 cup (250 g): GI= High, GL= High, Net carb= 28g

▤ Potato Soup, 1 cup (248 g): GI= High, GL= High, Net carb= 15g

▤ Pumpkin Pie, 1 slice (133 g): GI= High, GL= High, Net carb= 25g

▤ Pumpkin, canned, ½ cup (123 g): GI= High, GL= High, Net carb= 10g

▤ Roasted Butternut Squash, 1 cup (205 g): GI= High, GL= High, Net carb= 22g

▤ Roasted Parsnips, 1 cup (130 g): GI= High, GL= High, Net carb= 24g

▤ Roasted Sweet Potatoes, 1 cup (200 g): GI= High, GL= High, Net carb= 41g

▤ Scalloped Potatoes, 1 cup (245 g): GI= High, GL= High, Net carb= 32g

▤ Steamed White Corn, 1 cob (146 g): GI= High, GL= High, Net carb= 24g

▤ Stuffed Bell Peppers, with rice and meat, 1 pepper (200 g): GI= High, GL= High, Net carb= 35g

▤ Sweet and Sour Vegetables, 1 cup (150 g): GI= High, GL= High, Net carb= 32g

▤ Sweet Corn Ice Cream, ½ cup (86 g): GI= High, GL= High, Net carb= 21g

▤ Sweet Corn, boiled, 1 cob (146 g): GI= High, GL= High, Net carb= 24g

▤ Sweet Potato Casserole, 1 cup (200 g): GI= High, GL= High, Net carb= 37g

▤ Sweet Potato Fries, fast food, ½ cup (70 g): GI= High, GL= High, Net carb= 26g

▤ Sweet Potato Pie, 1 slice (125 g): GI= High, GL= High, Net carb= 42g

▤ Tater Tots, 1 cup (86 g): GI= High, GL= High, Net carb= 30g

▤ Vegetable Biryani, 1 cup (200 g): GI= High, GL= High, Net carb= 43g

▤ Vegetable Curry Puff, 1 puff (60 g): GI= High, GL= High, Net carb= 18g

▤ Vegetable Egg Rolls, 1 roll (80 g): GI= High, GL= High, Net carb= 15g

▤ Vegetable Fried Quinoa, 1 cup (200 g): GI= High, GL= High, Net carb= 45g

▤ Vegetable Fried Rice, 1 cup (140 g): GI= High, GL= High, Net carb= 40g

▤ Vegetable Korma, 1 cup (195 g): GI= High, GL= High, Net carb= 26g

▤ Vegetable Lasagna, 1 slice (200 g): GI= High, GL= High, Net carb= 25g

▤ Vegetable Lo Mein, 1 cup (200 g): GI= High, GL= High, Net carb= 44g

▤ Vegetable Paella, 1 cup (200 g): GI= High, GL= High, Net carb= 36g

▤ Vegetable Pizza, 1 slice (107 g): GI= High, GL= High, Net carb= 26g

▤ Vegetable Pot Pie, 1 pie (200 g): GI= High, GL= High, Net carb= 35g

▤ Vegetable Quiche, 1 slice (150 g): GI= High, GL= High, Net carb= 15g

▤ Vegetable Samosa, 1 piece (50 g): GI= High, GL= High, Net carb= 20g

▤ Vegetable Spring Roll, 2 rolls (80 g): GI= High, GL= High, Net carb= 24g

▤ Vegetable Stir Fry with Noodles, 1 cup (200 g): GI= High, GL= High, Net carb= 40g

▤ Vegetable Stuffed Pasta, 1 cup (150 g): GI= High, GL= High, Net carb= 40g

▤ Vegetable Tempura, 1 serving (130 g): GI= High, GL= High, Net carb= 18g

▤ Vegetarian Burger, 1 patty (100 g): GI= High, GL= High, Net carb= 15g

▤ Vegetarian Sausage, 1 link (75 g): GI= High, GL= High, Net carb= 12g

▤ Veggie Burrito, 1 burrito (200 g): GI= High, GL= High, Net carb= 47g

▤ Veggie Chips, 1 oz (28 g): GI= High, GL= High, Net carb= 15g

▤ Veggie Nuggets, 4 nuggets (60 g): GI= High, GL= High, Net carb= 18g

▤ Veggie Pasta, 1 cup (140 g): GI= High, GL= High, Net carb= 40g

▤ Veggie Potstickers, 6 pieces (170 g): GI= High, GL= High, Net carb= 40g

▤ Veggie Straws, 1 oz (28 g): GI= High, GL= High, Net carb= 15g

▤ Veggie Sushi Roll, 6 pieces (200 g): GI= High, GL= High, Net carb= 37g

ABOUT THE AUTHOR

"Dr. H. Maher" is a joint pen name under which Dr. Y. Naitlho, PharmD, and H. Naitlho, MS/MBA, co-write books.

Dr. Y. Naitlho PharmD has over 25 years of pharmacy practice, applied nutrition research, and writing. He is currently a pharmacist and health and nutrition writer. He is the author of several books in the field of food science and human nutrition, and applied nutrition.

Dr. Y. Naitlho received his Doctor of Pharmacy from Perm State Pharmaceutical Academy. As a pharmacist and nutrition professional, He ensures that book design meets readers' dynamic learning needs and that content meets reliability and integrity standards.

H. Naitlho has over 30 years of engineering practice and science and engineering Research. He is the author of several books in the field of business management and coauthor of numerous books in food science and human nutrition, food engineering, and applied nutrition.

H. Naitlho holds an Engineering degree from the École Supérieure d'Aéronautique et de l'Espace (Sup'Aéro), an Engineering degree from the École de l'Air (Salon de Provence) and has an MBA from Laureate International Universities, a post-graduate degree in Automatics from Paul Sabatier University, and a further post-graduate degree in Mechanics from Aix Marseille University.

H. Naitlho brings the engineering mindset and scientific rigor. He consistently refines ideas, analyzes data, and carries consistency and a great sense of detail to their work.

Made in the USA
Las Vegas, NV
28 February 2024

86428891R00207